mjgustxev 3/98

AORN PATIENT CLASSIFICATION INSTRUMENT FOR PERIOPERATIVE NURSING

Carol J. Applegeet, RN, MSN, CNOR, CNAA, FAAN

January, 1991
Revised, May 1993

Copyright © May, 1993. All rights reserved by
The Association of Operating Room Nurses, Inc.
2170 South Parker Road, Suite 300
Denver, Colorado 80231-5711

Printed in USA

ISBN 0-939583-83-6
MAN-046

CONTENTS

Preface Acknowledgements, v
  Dedication, vii

Chapter 1 **Introduction, 1**
  Overview of Publication, 1
  Historical Development of Instrument, 1

Chapter 2 **Review of the Literature, 3**

Chapter 3 **Research Methodology, 6**
  Purpose of the Study, 6
  Theoretical Basis of the Study, 6
  Background of the Study, 7
  Assumptions, 8
  Specific Aims of the Study, 8
  Definition of Terms, 8
  Summary of the Study, 8
  Study Limitations, 9
  Recommendations for Future Study, 10

Chapter 4 **AORN Patient Classification Instrument for Perioperative Nursing, 11**
  Instrument Description, 11
  The Instrument, 11
  Indicator Definitions, 16

Chapter 5 **Implementation of the Patient Classification Instrument in the Preoperative Setting, 18**
  Transport, 18
  Assessment, 19
  Medications, 20
  Comfort/Safety, 21
  Teaching, 22
  Procedures, 22
  Communication, 23
  Patient Condition, 23
  Preoperative Patient Acuity Categories, 24
  Samples of Preoperative Timing Activities, 24

Chapter 6 **Implementation of the Patient Classification Instrument in the Intraoperative Setting, 38**
  Suite Preparation, 38
  Patient Preparation, 39
  Surgical Procedure, 40
  Suite Clean Up, 40
  Intraoperative Acuity Categories, 41
  Common Problems in Computation, 42

Chapter 7 **Usefulness of the Instrument, 43**

Chapter 8 **Summary, 45**
  References, 45

Addendum **Blank Instrument Pages for Institutional Use, 47**

ACKNOWLEDGMENTS

Appreciation is extended to the many individuals who have contributed to the initial development of the AORN Patient Classification Instrument for Perioperative Nursing.

CONTRIBUTORS/REVIEWERS

Cynthia A. Bray, RN, MS, CNOR
Clinical Specialist
Hahnemann University Hospital
Philadelphia, Pennsylvania

Nell Crowder-Panten, RN, CNOR
Community Medical Center
Scranton, Pennsylvania

Elaine Thomson-Keith, RN, BSN, CNOR
Manager, Neurosensory OR/PACU
The Methodist Hospital
Houston, Texas

Susan Galczak Viola, RN, MS, CNOR
OR/PACU Coordinator
New Milford Hospital
New Milford, Connecticut

RESEARCH SITE COORDINATORS

John Price, RN, BSN, CNOR
Nurse Educator
Mississippi Baptist Medical Center
Jackson, Mississippi

Margery Sawyer, RN, BS, CNOR
Director, Surgical Services
Humana Hospital Gwinnett
Snellville, Georgia

RESEARCH SITES

Hahnemann University
Philadelphia, Pennsylvania

Humana Hospital Gwinnett
Snellville, Georgia

Jewish Hospital
Louisville, Kentucky

Outpatient Care Center
at Jewish Hospital
Louisville, Kentucky

Porter Memorial Hospital
Denver, Colorado

Saint Joseph Hospital
Denver, Colorado

Saint Mary's Hospital
Waterbury, Connecticut

San Jacinto Methodist Hospital
Bay Town, Texas

University of Mississippi
Jacksonville, Mississippi

University of Virginia
Charlottesville, Virginia

RESEARCH AGENCY

School of Nursing
Center for Nursing Research
University of Colorado
Health Sciences Center
Denver, Colorado

A. Sylvia Lewis, RN, PhD
Principal Investigator

Victoria Erickson, RN, PhD
Co-Investigator

Ruth Neil, RN, MS
Research Assistant

Special thanks are extended to the AORN Board of Directors for their foresight in providing the funds and support necessary for instrument development and the many members and AORN Headquarters staff on the Nursing Practices Committee who dreamed that such an instrument was useful and beneficial to the perioperative practitioners of today and tomorrow.

DEDICATION

This publication is dedicated to the members of the Association of Operating Room Nurses, Inc., whose excellence in practice contributes to the health care of our nation, with the hope that this instrument will prove both helpful and useful in preparing to meet the future of perioperative nursing practice.

CHAPTER 1
INTRODUCTION

Overview of Publication

By publishing the *AORN Patient Classification Instrument for Perioperative Nursing*, the Association of Operating Room Nurses, Inc., demonstrates its commitment to perioperative nursing practice. Individuals who choose to implement the tool in their own practice settings will find this publication useful. The intent of the publication is to provide the practitioner with a valid and reliable patient classification instrument designed specifically for the pre- and intraoperative phases of patient care and to assist with the implementation of a classification system in the perioperative setting. Successful implementation of a classification system requires a commitment by administration, nursing service, operating room (OR) management, and operating room staff. The instrument as presented may be modified by institutions to meet their own individual needs following validity and reliability studies.

The publication is divided into eight chapters. Chapter 1 is a historical review of the instrument's development including background information on the Association of Operating Room Nurses and perioperative nursing practice. The literature review in Chapter 2 provides a historical review of the development of patient classification systems, especially those specific to the operating room setting. The research summary of Chapter 3 includes the scientific framework of the instrument, study background, assumptions, aims and limitations, as well as definition of terms. Chapter 4 describes the instrument. Chapters 5 and 6 discuss the implementation of the instrument in the pre- and intraoperative phases respectively. Each chapter includes a description of the indicators of care and acuity categories. Chapter 7 describes the instrument's usefulness in the clinical setting. Chapter 8 includes the summary and references for the text.

Historical Development of the Instrument

This revised edition of the *AORN Patient Classification Instrument for Perioperative Nursing* has several changes. The tool has been modified slightly as the result of input from those who have utilized the instrument in their clinical settings. In addition, a second format for the tool has been developed. Both the original and revised formats are included in this printing. The AORN Philosophy has been revised from the 1988 edition. Finally, the research tools have been omitted from this printing. The entire research study is available by contacting the Association of Operating Room Nurses, Inc.

PHILOSOPHY OF THE ASSOCIATION OF OPERATING ROOM NURSES, INC.

The Association of Operating Room Nurses, Inc., is a voluntary organization of professional registered nurses concerned with perioperative patient care.

The Association believes nursing is a social institution that provides essential and significant health care services to meet evolving societal needs. The perioperative nurse uses knowledge, judgment, and skills based on the principles of physical, biological, physiological, behavioral, social and nursing science.

The Association believes that nurses must be ethical, responsible and accountable for quality patient care. The nurse engaged in perioperative nursing practice provides or facilitates care to surgical or other perioperative patients. The Association believes that research should be the foundation for perioperative nursing practice.

The Association believes that learning is a lifelong process and that perioperative nurses must assume responsibility for their ongoing education. The Association is committed to enabling perioperative nurses to meet that responsibility.

The Association believes that standards of nursing practice, interdisciplinary collaboration, and appropriate resource utilization enhance perioperative nursing practice.

The Association believes its activities should be structured to anticipate and meet society's perioperative health care needs.

PHILOSOPHY OF PERIOPERATIVE NURSING PRACTICE

The Philosophy of Perioperative Nursing Practice was developed and adopted by the AORN House of Delegates in February 1978. It was revised in November 1984, and again in March 1988. The abstracted philosophy states that the Association believes perioperative nursing derives its knowledge base from scientific principles that are integrated and applied through the nursing process. The patient, as the focal point of all nursing care activities, is entitled to quality, individualized care. Perioperative nursing is practiced in a highly technical, rapidly changing environment in which the continual addition of knowledge and skills by the practitioner is critical. While the perioperative nurse works in collaboration with other health professionals to determine and meet the patient's needs, the nurse has primary responsibility and accountability for nursing care of patients having surgical intervention. (*AORN Standards and Recommended Practices*, 1993).

AORN NURSING PRACTICES COMMITTEE

The Nursing Practices Committee was established by the AORN Board of Directors in 1981. In December 1983, the Nursing Practices Committee determined that development of a patient classification instrument should be its next project. Between December 1983 and January 1986, the work of the Nursing Practices Committee was directed toward other Association projects. The Committee did not begin work on the development of a patient classification instrument for perioperative nursing until 1986. On July 1, 1987, AORN contracted with the University of Colorado Center for Nursing Research, Denver, to assist in the development of a valid and reliable instrument for patient classification. In March 1989, members of the Nursing Practices Committee were retained as principle developers of the instrument; however, the Committee was renamed the Special Committee on Patient Classification Instrument for Perioperative Nursing. The charge to the Committee was to develop a valid and reliable patient classification instrument for perioperative nursing.

AORN publications were utilized throughout the development of the *AORN Patient Classification Instrument for Perioperative Nursing*. The *AORN Standards and Recommended Practices for Perioperative Nursing* served as the basis for development of the instrument. During the initial phases of development, the Committee reviewed the *Operating Room Staffing Study* (1985), *Competency Statements in Perioperative Nursing* (1989), and the *Surgical Experience: A Model for Professional Nursing Practice in the OR* (1978) for development of the instrument.

AORN GOALS AND STRATEGIES

The AORN Board of Directors approved a Strategic Plan in 1986. One goal of the strategic plan was to foster research. From 1987 to 1991, the Association identified implementation strategies within the research goal to support development and dissemination of the *AORN Patient Classification Instrument for Perioperative Nursing* and devoted funds for completion of the project.

AORN RESEARCH INITIATIVES

In April 1987, the AORN Board of Directors charged the AORN Research Committee to restructure the grants program. As a result, the AORN Research Policy Plan and Priority Statement and the AORN Clinical Research Grants Program were approved. The Policy Plan and Priority Statement identified classification of nursing practice phenomena specifically related to patient care as a priority.

CONCLUSION

The Special Committee on Patient Classification Instrument for Perioperative Nursing worked with the University of Colorado Center for Nursing Research to develop the classification instrument published here. It is the belief of the Committee that all appropriate Association materials and other relevant literature were utilized in development of the final instrument and that the instrument presented is both valid and reliable.

Publication and dissemination of the perioperative patient classification instrument is the culmination of a significant investment in time and energy by the Association of Operating Room Nurses, Inc., and is yet another mechanism to address the needs of the perioperative nursing community.

CHAPTER 2
REVIEW OF THE LITERATURE

The first recorded systematic observation and study of work was undertaken by Frederick W. Taylor in the late nineteenth century (Drucker, 1974). Workload analysis, however, was not used in hospitals nor was it used to assist nursing services until many years later.

Researchers have examined patient classification systems since the early 1960s. Originally designed to assist with the determination of nursing staffing, their current usefulness extends to budgeting, predictive modeling, and as part of methods to cost out nursing care. Classification systems were generally defined as the grouping of patients according to some observable or inferred characteristics. Patient classification is the identification of groups of patients to measure nursing care required.

Much is contained in the literature describing the end results of an ideal system. This system should: project staffing needs, match patient requirements with nursing resources, assist in justifying staffing patterns, and provide a basis for nursing charges. To accomplish these goals, the classification system selected must have application to the unit. In specialty nursing, the unique characteristics of that area can make application of existing systems difficult, therefore, some specialty areas have developed their own instruments.

The two methods used in instrument design are prototype and factor evaluation. The prototype method classifies patients by matching actual patient characteristics with those in preestablished categories. They are then matched to the appropriate category description. Difficulties with this design relate to establishing acceptable reliability because of the broad categories. Factor evaluation design delineates specific elements of care that are critical indicators of care for the setting. These elements are combined to form a scoring system. Even though this design is more reliable, it also may be more time-consuming to complete (Giovannetti, 1979). Studies conducted by Verran (1986) indicated that most newly developed classification systems use the factor evaluation method because of its higher interobserver reliability. Use of standards of care, nursing diagnosis, and risk indicators and assessment factors enabled development of a patient classification system that utilized both designs. This hybrid system was incorporated into the quality assurance program and is part of the permanent documentation on the hospital record (McNeal, Hutelmyer & Abrami, 1987).

In spite of the numerous studies conducted on classification systems, there is a continuing mistrust by staff nurses and nursing management alike of the established system. For example, Audette and Tilquin (1977) determined a need for inclusion on indirect care and tasks unrelated to patients in determining workload for nurses. They also stressed the importance of building psychological care into the system. Giovannetti (1979) emphasized the importance of utilizing nursing care time as a rational approach for looking at workload. This investigator noted that many patient classification systems are based on unidimensional and partial assessment of patient care requirements and quantifications based on existing practice. These classification systems, therefore, should not be used to "lock in" staffing and budgetary concerns. Establishing and maintaining reliability and validity of a patient classification system is imperative if the system is to be accepted. In a study by Giovannetti and Mayer (1984), predictive validity of a classification instrument was tested by comparing prospective ratings of care needs with retrospective reports of actual care provided. Percent agreement scores were used to measure the comparison. Overall prediction of exact patient care was 79%. There is need for further study in this area to look at adequacy of staffing patterns and percent of activities that are unpredictable in certain clinical settings, such as intensive care units (Whitney & Killien, 1987).

Williams (1988) explored the methodology of validating existing patient classification systems as an alternative to internal development. Williams described preliminary appraisal method, such as similar types of units, and the ability of the instrument to be generalized to different populations. Once initial feasibility is determined, content validity must be established. This is accomplished by obtaining the judgment of experts (eg, experi-

Review of the Literature

enced staff nurses) regarding the accuracy and adequacy of the indicators of care. After content validity has been established by expert practitioners, the next step is to obtain criterion related validity. This type of validity can be either concurrent or predictive. Use of validity testing on existing patient classification systems can offer an alternative to costly development of new systems. An effective classification system can offer nurse administrators and practicing clinicians many benefits. The data generated by classification systems give managers valuable instruments for planning, budgeting, and marketing and can be used to monitor quality of care.

Patient classification systems also have been developed for establishing staffing guidelines. These systems can be utilized for determination and allocation of nursing resources to effectively meet the demands of the patient population. Because nursing services are the largest users of personnel, nursing administration must be able to justify staff expenses. The greatest challenge is not only determining how much staff should be employed, but also providing the number of qualified staff to meet patient care requirements on a day-to-day and shift-by-shift basis.

The effectiveness of nursing care not only depends on the caregiver, but also on the condition of the patient. Patient classification systems assist in resource allocation that encompass characteristics of both the nurse and patient. The assignment of a nurse to a patient is the basic operational unit that identifies cost and quality of nursing care. The optimum decision assigns the most competent nurse to the most complex patient. Complex patients demand a high level of skill and more time. Thus, cost reimbursement for nursing care must consider the nurse provider and the complexity of the care delivered. In addition to staffing, patient classification systems also assist nurse managers in costing out nursing services. A more equitable distribution of costs, which assigns the charge to the patient who is receiving the services, is possible. Classification systems are an essential first step to demonstrate and quantify the standard of nursing care being delivered. Classification systems allow the manager to predict when supplemental staffing in the unit is necessary. This affords all patients safe and optimum care. It should be noted, however, that many of these instruments document nursing activities related to a standard, and it cannot be assumed that the patient outcome is actually reflected. For example, Trofino (1989) used hospitals accredited by the Joint Commission on Accreditation of Healthcare Organizations (JCAHO) in a study of the relationship of nursing care hours to length of stay per diagnosis related group (DRG). This relationship implies certain staffing patterns and a defined set of parameters for quality and appropriateness of care (JCAHO, 1992). The actual measurement of patient care quality, however, cannot be accomplished with the patient classification system.

The introduction of the Prospective Payment System, which utilizes DRGs for hospital reimbursement, has accelerated activity to separate out the cost of nursing care. DRGs have forced nurse executives to look seriously at capturing the diminishing dollar and to convert patient care units revenue into producing cost centers (Covaleski, 1981; Higgerson, & Van Slyck, 1982).

In 1983, Curtin advocated the development of 23 nursing care categories to determine the cost of nursing services per DRG. To separate the nursing component of the care and the treatment process for DRGs, Curtin proposed that a nursing care strategy be developed for each of the 467 DRGs. Within each DRG, nursing care would be assessed using a patient classification system. Since 1983, there have been increasing numbers of hospital and nurse administrators who have proposed differing methods for allocating nursing costs to the DRG cost center.

A comprehensive nursing intensity index developed by Reitz was intended to assist nursing in standardizing patient classification related to DRGs (Reitz, 1985). Despite these efforts, a study by Nagaprasanna in 1988 found that 40% of patient classification systems were internally developed. According to Nagaprasanna (1988), the exact number of classification systems is unknown. Many systems were designed to measure inpatient acute care units. Few are oriented toward specialty units such as ambulatory care units, operating rooms, and postanesthesia care units (PACU).

Outpatient and emergency room classification systems have been developed by Verran (1986); Horn, Buckle, and Carver (1988); and Helmer, Freitas, and Onaha (1988).

A patient classification system for the PACU was described by Shirk and Marion (1986). This system classified patients according to the time they spent in PACU as well as nursing function. This instrument utilized six classes. Classes one to four have a predetermined length of stay in PACU. Classes five and six designate a nurse to patient ratio as well as final destination after discharge from PACU. All classes reflect nursing care in minutes.

In an effort to bring the operating room into a similar format as that of a hospital-wide system under development, a factor-evaluation instrument was designed by Girard and Keeler (1986). They found that the needs of the operating room were entirely different from the rest of the hospital. These authors developed an instrument that utilized six categories and assigned points in each category. Number of personnel assigned to the room was decided by use of the points assigned. Personnel hours were determined by multiplying number of personnel by projected time for each procedure assigned. The type of personnel needed for each procedure was not addressed.

The operating room is a specialty area in which intensity of nursing care can be assessed by factors other than case load. Hart (1985) described a classification system that utilized four acuity levels. These levels were based on cost of services and type of surgery. Four levels were utilized ranging from minimum setup through procedures requiring four or more operating room personnel, special rooms, and/or maximum use of specialized sutures.

A patient classification system has been described by Parrinello (1987) for use in ambulatory surgery settings. The instrument used 35 indicators of care, which were descriptive of potential nursing needs. The indicators were divided into four groups by type of nursing intervention. These included assessment/observation needs, functional needs, nursing intervention needs, and special needs. Each indicator had an assigned weight based on the relative intensity of the nursing activities. By totaling weights, patients were classified into one of four categories of nursing intensity. The acuity categories had preassigned nursing care hour requirements. Nursing interventions related only to the pre- and postoperative phases.

The literature review revealed there have been few attempts to develop an OR classification instrument for use in both inpatient and ambulatory surgery settings. Although these instruments were designed for unit-specific settings, there are no instruments developed for use in a variety of settings.

In summary, in an era of increasingly sophisticated and complex health care delivery systems, classification instruments serve several purposes. Classification systems can document patient requirements for nursing care, document shifts in patient requirements, help project staffing needs, and document costs for nursing care provided. The literature describes the importance and difficulty of developing a classification system in specialty areas.

CHAPTER 3
RESEARCH METHODOLOGY

Purpose of the Study

AORN demonstrates an ongoing commitment to maintaining its standards of perioperative nursing practice. Therefore, the patient classification instrument for perioperative nursing was developed to provide guidelines for resource allocation so that these standards can be met in a cost-effective manner.

Patients have always been classified in some manner. Historically, this was according to their diagnosis, age, and/or sex. Anesthesiologists have utilized classes for documenting severity of illness as well as for billing purposes. More recently, sophisticated patient classification systems have been developed and used by patient care units. Their purpose is to provide staffing patterns, which are consistent with the types and numbers of patients, the severity of illnesses, and/or nursing care required. Nursing managers, in an effort to justify and accurately predict staffing needs as well as monitor productivity levels, utilize classification information to deal with cost control and budgetary process. In addition, JCAHO mandated nursing departments to define, implement, and maintain a system for determining demonstrated patient needs, appropriate nursing interventions, and priority of care.

The introduction of Prospective Payment Systems for hospital reimbursement accelerated activity to explicate cost of nursing care. Patient classification systems can be integrated into nursing management programs that compliment the DRG Medical Management System.

More recently, on a very limited scale, patient classification systems have been developed for the operating room. These systems vary in structure, but have patient charging as their main focus. These charges include personnel utilization and supply/equipment needs. Little or no consideration has been given to patient acuity or the level of nursing care required.

Patient classification systems are instruments designed to measure direct and indirect nursing time required to care for individual patients. The classification system for perioperative nursing allocates the cost of surgery to the patient receiving the actual care.

The purpose of the research study undertaken by AORN and the University of Colorado Center for Nursing Research was to develop a patient classification instrument that would provide a valid and reliable data base for cost identification of nursing services.

Theoretical Basis of the Study

The nursing process and general systems theory were used as the organizing framework for development of the patient classification instrument.

Perioperative nursing currently utilizes the nursing process as a practice framework. Therefore, it was apparent that the instrument also should reflect the nursing process components of perioperative nursing practice. These nursing process components served to identify the critical indicators of care activities that universally occur throughout the patient's surgical experience.

Nursing utilizes systematic observational and problem-solving techniques to identify potential problems and appropriate interventions and to evaluate the effectiveness of the interventions. The nursing process describes this method, and through its components, sets nursing process into motion. The nursing process is pivotal, therefore, to perioperative nursing and to the instrument's design.

AORN "Standards of perioperative nursing practice" were used to conceptually define the instrument's indicators of care. Timing studies were conducted in a variety of surgical settings to establish weights for the indicators and to set classification categories. This approach was based on two assumptions. First, the surgical services used as data collection sites for this study had an adequate level of staff to provide safe nursing care and second, nursing staff practiced in accordance with standards required for JCAHO accreditation.

Another basis of the study was to view a patient classification system as part of a broader systems model designed for cost identification of nursing services, congruent with other authors (Higgerson & Van Slyck, 1982; Sovie & Smith, 1986). Using a systems approach, Van Slyck (1987) viewed patient classification systems as one of five interdependent and interrelated systems. These systems were: 1) a belief system or philosophical framework that identifies the organization's beliefs as they relate to nursing care; 2) a patient classification system that categorizes patients into distinct groups based on preestablished criteria; 3) a staffing system that delivers service based on qualified acuity of patients; 4) a costing system that delineates nursing costs for each patient, and 5) an audit system that formally and systematically verifies patient acuity levels. Thus, the development of a patient classification system for perioperative nursing was seen as only one component of a model designed to identify costs of delivered services so that health care can be effectively managed.

Concepts from the general systems theory contributed to the organizational framework. The general systems theory views the individual patient holistically as a "open" system. Life is maintained at a steady state through continuous input-transformation-feedback process.

Within perioperative nursing the patient is viewed as a system, and the nurse functions to assist the patient in maintaining a steady state. Nursing interaction becomes the link between environmental/physical/psychological changes and patient adaptation. The goal of perioperative nursing is, therefore, to enhance the adaptive level of the individual through a systematic method of practice—the nursing process.

Background of the Study

Some major decisions were made during the process of conceptualizing an instrument to measure the amount of nursing care received by a patient during the perioperative experience. First, the boundaries were defined wherein perioperative care was delivered. Initially, preoperative, intraoperative, and postoperative phases were identified; reconsideration of the postoperative phase (vis-a-vis postanesthesia care unit standards of care) led to the decision to focus on patient acuity in the preoperative and intraoperative phases only.

Second, a time-based factor evaluation system was selected. The prototype (profile) or factor evaluation patient classification system will determine in part the degree of reliability and validity obtained. Prototype systems are more global and tend to obscure nursing activities. In contrast, factor evaluation systems contain a number of separate and weighted elements of the domain of nursing care actions. Although a factor evaluation system requires more detailed decision making by the nurse, this type of system has a distinct advantage in that it lends itself to precise validity and reliability testing (Hinshaw & Atwood, 1983). In line with this, the perioperative patient classification instrument measures acuity of adult patients (ie, 18 years and older) who undergo surgery in both inpatient and ambulatory settings as well as preoperative and intraoperatove patient acuity. The instrument also measures services delivered and not "perceived care needs." The instrument's content was developed to include psychosocial interventions, such as patient or family teaching, anticipatory guidance and emotional support, and chronic conditions that affect overall care.

Finally, the instrument reflects components of the nursing process. Halloran (1985) stated that nursing is as much an intellectual endeavor as it is a physical one and criticized the task-oriented nature of most patient classification systems that do no recognize nursing assessment and evaluation. Van Slyck (1987) concurred with Halloran's position and indicated that the development of a patient classification system in the context of the nursing process provided a more accurate identification of nursing services.

In addition to the above decisions and considerations, certain issues related to patient classification systems were addressed. Vaughan and MacLeod (1980) recommended that nursing organizations take the lead in developing and promoting the use of standard definitions, classifications, and time figures for nursing care. These authors indicated that money is better spent on improving methodology, rather than each institution working independently. In contrast, several investigators have taken a different position. That is, in order to establish a valid patient classification system, time studies must be carried out in each hospital due to variations in environment, ancillary support, and nursing routines (McKubbin, 1985; Sovie, 1985; Van Slyck, 1985; Vanpulte, 1985). The methodology employed in this study combines elements of both positions. The Association of Operating Room Nurses took the initiative to sponsor the development of a patient classification system for perioperative nursing.

Assumptions

This study was based on the following assumptions:
1. Perioperative nursing standards are consistent across sites.
2. Perioperative nursing activities can be observed.
3. Perioperative nursing activities can be measured.
4. Perioperative nursing activities can be classified.

Specific Aims of the Study

1. To identify and describe indicators of perioperative nursing care.
2. To assign weights to these indicators and determine patient acuity categories.
3. To establish content and criterion validity of the instrument.
4. To establish interrater reliability and generalizability of the instrument.

Definition of Terms

Perioperative Nursing Practice

Conceptual Definition. The performance of nursing activities in the preoperative, intraoperative, and postoperative phases of the patient's surgical experience.

Operational Definition. The performance of direct and delegated nursing activities occurring in the preoperative and intraoperative phases of the patient's experience.

Preoperative Phase

Conceptual Definition. Begins when the decision for surgical intervention is made and ends with transference of the patient to the operating room bed.

Operational Definition. Begins with the patient to the preoperative/holding area or upon arrival of the patient in the preoperative/holding area and ends when the operating room nurse assumes responsibility.

Intraoperative Phase

Conceptual Definition. Begins when the patient is transferred to the operating room bed and ends when he/she is admitted to the postanesthesia care area.

Operational Definition. Begins when the operating room nurse assumes responsibility of the patient and ends when suite clean up has been completed.

Patient Classification

The categorization of patients according to some assessment of their nursing care requirements over a specified period of time (Giovannetti, 1979).

Indicators of Care

The most frequently occurring direct and indirect nursing care activities provided to patients during the perioperative period.

Direct Nursing Care

All "hands on" activities including patient/family education and emotional support necessary in delivery of care to patients (Curtin, 1983).

Indirect Nursing Care

Activities related to nursing care other than "hands on" (ie, charting, collaboration, suite preparation).

Delegated Nursing Care

Technical functions provided by other healthcare individuals at the direction of the registered nurse.

Summary of the Study

The primary purpose of this study was to develop and estimate the reliability and validity of a perioperative classification instrument. The term perioperative was defined, for this study, to include the preoperative and intraoperative phases of a patient's surgical experience. A factor evaluation instrument was designed to measure adult patient acuity in terms of nursing care provided. The instrument was developed through a process that included four stages. Each stage was delineated by a specific research aim and related questions. The aims encompassed the following: 1) identification and conceptual description of the major indicators and concomitant nursing activities. This was accomplished by a panel of experts, a questionnaire survey, and clinical validation; 2) timing studies conducted in six institutions' operating rooms to determine weights of the preoperative nursing activities and intraoperative indicators and the respective acuity categories; 3) construction of an original instrument and establishment of content and concurrent validity; and 4) estimation of interrater reliability and generalizability of the instrument in four institutions and construction of the final form of the instrument.

The instrument's design was structured to measure preoperative and intraoperative acuity separately. The preoperative component contains seven nursing activity domains: patient transport, assessment, medications, procedures, teaching, safety and comfort measures, and communication. Each of these domains consist of specific weight time-based activities. An additional item that reflected a patient's health condition was included in the instrument's content. Preoperative patient acuity was partitioned into three categories based on amount of nursing care delivered.

The intraoperative component of the instrument consists of four indicators: suite preparation, patient preparation, surgical procedure, and suite clean up. Each indicator is divided into time levels and each level is assigned a weight that reflects the empirical mean for that level. Six acuity categories are established for the intraoperative component of the instrument.

The instrument's content and weights were reevaluated and confirmed by a panel of experts, four groups of perioperative nurses who participated in the reliability study, and by repeated timings on specific activities that were questioned by the nurses. Good concurrent validity (r=.714) was obtained for the intraoperative acuity categories by comparing the instrument classification performance with experts' rankings in a sample of 150 different surgical procedures. Moderate size correlation coefficients were attained for patient preparations, surgical procedure, and suite clean up. This finding, however, did not apply to the freestanding surgery center. Interrater reliability, assessed by an average percentage of agreement, was quite high. The average agreement across preoperative activities was 97.8%; for the intraoperative indicator, agreement was 93.4%. A more critical measure of reliability was the assignment of patients to acuity categories. The raters in the preoperative area agreed 100% on this variable, and intraoperative raters reached 92.2% agreement. To ascertain the amount of variance in patients' scores due to interrater performance, a generalizability study was conducted. Coefficients of .99 and .98 were obtained for the preoperative and intraoperative acuity scores respectively. Sites and patients within sites had the largest variance contributions. A complete review of the instrument was conducted at the end of the study by a panel of experts and investigators. A final form of the instrument was then constructed.

Some salient features of the instrument were identified during the course of the study. The very low and nonsignificant correlations obtained between preoperative nursing time and nursing time of the intraoperative indicators (for five of the six sites) lends support for two separate acuity measures. Sites varied in the number of different preoperative nursing activities and indicate a need to expand or contract the inventory of activities to fit the setting. The weights assigned to the various time levels for each intraoperative indicator allowed for more specificity as to the distribution of nursing time for the entire intraoperative period. Two patients may be assigned to the same acuity category, but indicator weights may differ. This variation would have implications for justifying staffing needs as well as identifying costs.

Study Limitations

Limitations of the study were related to the types of samples used, when the data were collected, and the method used in data collection. The study used a convenience sample of sites and patients. The sample size for each site in the timed study (n=50-86) also limited the validity of the findings. Data were collected consecutively over a 2 to 3 month period in each site and the time of year for data collection by site (ie, spring, summer, and fall months). The volunteer status of the data collectors also influenced the selection of patients who were entered in the study. The days on which data collection occurred was dependent on whether the data collector could devote time to this activity. Very few emergency surgeries and no trauma cases were included in the timed sample. Data obtained from a large, representative sample over a longer period would lend more credibility to the findings.

Another limitation of the study was its national scope. Although having different types of facilities located in different geographical areas may be viewed as a strength, the distance between investigator and collection sites posed some difficulties. It hindered close monitoring of the data collection process and caused delays in problem solving or providing clarification of procedures. The method of data collection posed another validity threat, in interaction between observer and subject. Although nursing staffs were informed of the study, the effect of being observed (especially when the observer has a stopwatch in hand) on individual behavior is well known (Mitchell, 1979). In some cases being timed was interpreted to mean, "how fast can I do..." or "my performance is being critically reviewed." Although feedback on the presence was not a problem, potential for different performance existed.

Recommendations for Future Study

1. Increase the data base of the timed activities.
2. Develop studies to estimate concurrent validity of the preoperative and intraoperative classification categories using the criterion of nursing staffing patterns and workload.
3. Implement further study to estimate the instrument's validity in freestanding surgery centers.
4. Determine commonalities and differences in patient acuity among various institutions (eg, public teaching hospitals vs private/for-profit hospitals).
5. Identify nursing staff costs relative to surgery DRGs.
6. Describe shifts in institutional perioperative acuity (eg, trends, patterns) and their impact on staffing patterns.
7. Develop a subjective (qualitative) instrument to measure perioperative nursing complexity (eg, magnitude estimation techniques). This would complement the classification instrument that is based on time requirements only.
8. Develop a classification instrument for pediatric surgery patients.

CHAPTER 4
AORN PATIENT CLASSIFICATION INSTRUMENT FOR PERIOPERATIVE NURSING

Implementation of the perioperative classification system in the clinical setting requires an investment in time, energy, and resources. As presented, the instrument is valid and reliable. Those who wish to modify the instrument to meet individual institutional needs will need to conduct reliability and validity studies prior to alteration of the instrument. In the event that validity and reliability studies are not conducted, when alterations are made in the tool, the accuracy of the acuity data may be in question.

It is possible to implement the tool in sections, that is, only the preoperative or only the intraoperative acuity depending on the needs of the institution. It is suggested that prior to implementation of the classification system several factors be reviewed.

First, review the summary of the research conducted to provide a valid and reliable instrument, which is contained in the proceeding chapters of this text. Second, become familiar with the definition of the indicators (see page 16), noted on the instrument and the accompanying weights. An abbreviated list of the definitions can be found on (page 16). Thirdly, review the acuity categories noted for the preoperative and intraoperative phases. All staff members responsible for utilizing the instrument must be familiar with each of these steps and must be comfortable in implementing the tool. Prior to implementation, the institution should determine the expected uses of the instrument.

Modifications made in the instrument will require expected extensive study and research. In the event that some preoperative indicators or activities are not applicable in a particular setting, acuity categories will need to be modified accordingly.

Instrument Description

Either of the two formats for the Patient Classification Instrument included in this section, pages 12 and 13 or 14 and 15, can be utilized in the clinical setting. The original format, pages 12 and 13, places the pre- and intraoperative indicators and weights on the front side of the page with descriptive information on the reverse. The second format, pages 14 and 15, suggested by those who have implemented the tool in the clinical setting, places the preoperative indicators, weights, and descriptions on the facing page and the intraoperative indicators, weights, and descriptions of the reverse. The modified format allows the user to complete either the preoperative or the intraoperative sections without turning the tool over for reference.

Beneath each of the indicator columns are acuity categories determined to be valid for this particular tool within the context of the research study completed. A space has been left for the identifying data for each patient.

At the top of the instrument, there is space for completion of the surgical procedure and the admission status of the patient.

Nursing personnel familiar with the instrument, its definitions, and acuity categories can complete the scoring in five minutes or less per patient. The instrument is easily completed by imprinting the patient information in the section marked "patient data," noting the patient's admission status, indicating the surgical procedure, and scoring the indicators according to the definitions. The scores are circled, or in the situations where the factor may be multiplied by the number of nursing care occurrences, they are calculated. The subtotal scores then are added to determine the total score. The total score determines the acuity category. Nursing personnel may be needed to score the instrument, but they are not required to compute the totals and determine the acuity categories. This could be completed by a clerk or by a computer program.

Scoring should be done concurrently to assure accuracy of the data; however, some facilities score the tool retrospectively using charted data. Use of retrospective data may skew the final acuity categories because of incomplete documentation of nursing activities.

The admission status has been divided into three categories: outpatient, AM, and inpatient.

Admission Status:
Outpatient, AM, Inpatient
Procedure: _____

AORN PATIENT CLASSIFICATION

Preoperative

Transport

Floor/Unit	4
Floor/Unit with monitor	8
Intensive Care unit	8
Floor/Unit special bed	12
Outpatient	0

Assessment

Routine	2
Routine with monitor	3
Extensive	4

Medications

IM injection	1 × ____ =
Add to IV bag	1 × ____ =
IV fluid administration	2 × ____ =
IV meds (push)	2 × ____ =
Eye meds	4
	Subtotal

Comfort/Safety

Secure belongings	1 × ____ =
Help change position	1 × ____ =
Assist with elimination	1 × ____ =
Emotional support (patient/family)	1 × ____ =
Constant monitoring	8
	Subtotal

Teaching

Routine re: surgery (patient or family)	1
Discharge/Home care (patient or family)	2
	Subtotal

Procedures

Skin prep: (limb)	1
Skin prep: (trunk)	2
Assist A-line	3
Assist breast measurement	3
Fetal monitoring	5
Epidural blocks	6
Axillary blocks	4
	Subtotal

Communication

Charting-add data	1
-extensive	2
Collaboration	1
	Subtotal

Patient Condition

Disability (blind, deaf, communication barrier, cognitive, foreign lang)	2

Preoperative Acuity Categories

Total Pre op score _____
Circle one:
7 or less	Category I
8 to 10	Category II
11 +	Category III

Intraoperative

Suite Preparation

Minor	1
Standard	2
Major	3
Extensive	6

Patient Preparation

Minor	2
Standard	3
Major	5
Extensive I	7
Extensive II	14

Surgical Procedure

Minor	4
Standard	7
Major	12
Extensive I	20
Extensive II	33
Extensive III	58

Suite Clean Up

Standard	1
Major	2
Extensive	4

Intraoperative Acuity Categories

Total Intra op score _____
Circle one:
8	Category I
9 to 20	Category II
21 to 29	Category III
30 to 44	Category IV
45 to 64	Category V
65+	Category VI

Patient Data

Version 9

4/92

Admission Status: Circle type of patient outpatient, (AM) patient admitted day of surgery, or inpatient.

Transport: Identification of patient, determination of appropriate method of transport, and transport accomplished. Varies according to presence of patient support equipment (monitors, suctions, IV's) and location of hospital unit.

Assessment: *Routine*-History and physical, verification of procedure, review of patient record and documentation. *Routine with monitor*-Routine assessment/monitor in place. *Extensive*- Routine assessment/extensive may have monitor.

Medications: *PO, IM, IV fluids, add to IV, IV push*-Includes preparation, administration, evaluation, and charting. If more than one, multiply number by assigned weight. *Eye medications*-Includes instillation, monitoring, evaluation, and charting.

Comfort/Safety: *Secure belongings*-Assistance with undressing, identification and placement of belongings. *Help change position*-General comfort measurers (blanket, pillow, position change). Multiply by weight of 1. *Assist with elimination*-Assist to bathroom or use of bedpan/urinal. Multiply by weight of 1. *Emotional support*- Support given not accompanied by other activities. Multiply by weight of 1. *Constant monitoring*- Constant one-to-one ratio of care.

Teaching: *Routine*-Patient/family teaching including content related to surgical procedure not accompanied by other activities. *Discharge/Home Care*-Routine plus content related to discharge planning/home care.

Procedures: *Skin prep*-Preparation, skin shave, equipment disposal, and charting for preps performed on limbs/trunks. *Assist with A-line, breast measurement, fetal monitoring*-Procurement, preparation, assistance with procedure, disposal of equipment, and charting. *Epidural and axillary blocks*-Procurement, preparation, assistance with procedure, disposal of equipment, evaluation, and charting.

Communication: *Charting, additional data*-Recording additional information, beyond that associated with other activities. *Charting, extensive*-Ongoing progress notes, and additional orders. *Collaboration*-Communicating/consulting with others regarding changes in patient status/situational problems.

Patient Condition: Patients with physical or mental disability, communication barrier, and/or debilitated/frail elderly.

Suite Preparation: Obtaining positioning equipment, establishing/maintaining a sterile field. Suite prep calculated by subtracting (-) time suite prep began from time patient arrives in OR times (×) number of nursing personnel.

Level	Weight	Ranges (minutes)	
Minor	1	15 or less	Time patient arrives in OR
Standard	2	16-30	-Time suite prep began
Major	3	31-45	(minutes) × number of nursing personnel
Extensive	6	46 or greater	

Patient Preparation: Reconfirming patient identity, surgical procedure, consent; positioning; monitoring; preparing incision site; emotional support; comfort/safety; assist with induction; creating/maintaining sterile field; and monitoring the environment. Patient prep is calculated by subtracting (-) time patient arrived in OR from time incision made times (×) number of nursing personnel.

Level	Weight	Ranges (minutes)	
Minor	2	30 or less	
Standard	3	31-45	Time incision made
Major	5	46-75	-Time patient arrives in OR
Extensive I	7	76-105	(minutes) × number of nursing personnel
Extensive II	14	106 or greater	

Surgical Procedure: Total time patient is undergoing procedure. Surgical procedure calculated by subtracting (-) the incision time from the time patient leaves OR times (×) number of nursing personnel.

Level	Weight	Ranges (minutes)	
Minor	4	60 or less	
Standard	7	61-105	
Major	12	106-180	Time patient leaves OR
Extensive I	20	181-300	-Time incision made
Extensive II	33	301-495	(minutes) × number of nursing personnel
Extensive III	58	496 or greater	

Suite Clean Up: *Standard*-All activities involved in decontamination of suite; supplies and equipment requisition; and equipment transport and restocking. *Major*-Standard with specialized equipment and/or microscopes and moderate body fluid/blood spillage. *Extensive*-Standard with extensive equipment (6 or more sets), or extensive radical surgery. Suite clean up is calculated by subtracting (-) the time the patient leaves the OR from the time of completion of the suite clean up times (×) number of nursing personnel.

Level	Weight	Ranges (minutes)	
Standard	1	15 or less	Time suite clean up complete
Major	2	16-30	-Time patient leaves OR
Extensive	4	31 or greater	(minutes) × number of nursing personnel

AORN PATIENT CLASSIFICATION
Preoperative

Admission Status:
Outpatient, AM, Inpatient
Procedure: _____

Transport

Floor/Unit	4
Floor/Unit with monitor	8
Intensive Care unit	8
Floor/Unit special bed	12
Outpatient	0

Assessment

Routine	2
Routine with monitor	3
Extensive	4

Medications

IM injection	1 × ____ =
Add to IV bag	1 × ____ =
IV fluid administration	2 × ____ =
IV meds (push)	2 × ____ =
Eye meds	4
	Subtotal

Comfort/Safety

Secure belongings	1 × ____ =
Help change position	1 × ____ =
Assist with elimination	1 × ____ =
Emotional support (patient/family)	1 × ____ =
Constant monitoring	8
	Subtotal

Teaching

Routine re: surgery (patient or family)	1
Discharge/Home care (patient or family)	2
	Subtotal

Procedures

Skin prep: (limb)	1
Skin prep: (trunk)	2
Assist A-line	3
Assist breast measurement	3
Fetal monitoring	5
Epidural blocks	6
Axillary blocks	4
	Subtotal

Communication

Charting-add data	1
-extensive	2
Collaboration	1
	Subtotal

Patient Condition

Disability (blind, deaf, communication barrier, cognitive, foreign lang)	2

Preoperative Acuity Categories

Total Pre op score _____
Circle one:
- 7 or less — Category I
- 8 to 10 — Category II
- 11 + — Category III

Admission Status: Circle type of patient outpatient, (AM) patient admitted day of surgery, or inpatient.

Transport: Identification of patient, determination of appropriate method of transport, and transport accomplished. Varies according to presence of patient support equipment (monitors, suctions, IV's) and location of hospital unit.

Assessment: *Routine*-History and physical, verification of procedure, review of patient record and documentation. *Routine with monitor*-Routine assessment/monitor in place. *Extensive*-Routine assessment/extensive may have monitor.

Medications: *PO, IM, IV fluids, add to IV, IV push*-Includes preparation, administration, evaluation, and charting. If more than one, multiply number by assigned weight. *Eye medications*-Includes instillation, monitoring, evaluation, and charting.

Comfort/Safety: *Secure belongings*-Assistance with undressing, identification, and placement of belongings. *Help change position*-General comfort measurers (blanket, pillow, position change). Multiply by weight of 1. *Assist with elimination*-Assist to bathroom or use of bedpan/urinal. Multiply by weight of 1. *Emotional support*-Support given not accompanied by other activities. Multiply by weight of 1. *Constant monitoring*-Constant one-to-one ratio of care.

Teaching: *Routine*- Patient/family teaching including content related to surgical procedure not accompanied by other activities. *Discharge/Home Care*-Routine plus content related to discharge planning/home care.

Procedures: *Skin prep*-Preparation, skin shave, equipment disposal, and charting for preps performed on limbs/trunks. *Assist with A-line, breast measurement, fetal monitoring*-Procurement, preparation, assistance with procedure, disposal of equipment, and charting. *Epidural and axillary blocks*-Procurement, preparation, assistance with procedure, disposal of equipment, evaluation, and charting.

Communication: *Charting, additional data*-Recording additional information, beyond that associated with other activities. *Charting, extensive*-Ongoing progress notes, and additional orders. *Collaboration*-Communicating/consulting with others regarding changes in patient status/situational problems.

Patient Condition: Patients with physical or mental disability, communication barrier, and/or debilitated/frail elderly.

Patient Data
Version 9
4/92

AORN PATIENT CLASSIFICATION
Intraoperative

Admission Status:
Outpatient, AM, Inpatient
Procedure: _____
_____

Suite Preparation	
Minor	1
Standard	2
Major	3
Extensive	6

Patient Preparation	
Minor	2
Standard	3
Major	5
Extensive I	7
Extensive II	14

Surgical Procedure	
Minor	4
Standard	7
Major	12
Extensive I	20
Extensive II	33
Extensive III	58

Suite Clean Up	
Standard	1
Major	2
Extensive	4

Intraoperative Acuity Categories	
Total Intra op score _____	
Circle one:	
8	Category I
9 to 20	Category II
21 to 29	Category III
30 to 44	Category IV
45 to 64	Category V
65+	Category VI

Patient Data

Suite Preparation: Obtaining positioning equipment, establishing/maintaining a sterile field. Suite prep calculated by subtracting (-) time suite prep began from time patient arrives in OR times (x) number of nursing personnel.

Level	Weight	Ranges (minutes)
Minor	1	15 or less
Standard	2	16-30
Major	3	31-45
Extensive	6	46 or greater

Patient Preparation: Reconfirming patient identity, surgical procedure, consent; positioning; monitoring; preparing incision site; emotional support; comfort/safety; assist with induction; creating/maintaining sterile field; and monitoring the environment. Patient prep is calculated by subtracting (-) time patient arrived in OR from time incision made times (x) number of nursing personnel.

Level	Weight	Ranges (minutes)
Minor	2	30 or less
Standard	3	31-45
Major	5	46-75
Extensive I	7	76-105
Extensive II	14	106 or greater

Surgical Procedure: Total time patient is undergoing procedure. Surgical procedure calculated by subtracting (-) the incision time from the time patient leaves OR times (x) number of nursing personnel.

Level	Weight	Ranges (minutes)
Minor	4	60 or less
Standard	7	61-105
Major	12	106-180
Extensive I	20	181-300
Extensive II	33	301-495
Extensive III	58	496 or greater

Suite Clean Up: *Standard*-All activities involved in decontamination of suite, supplies and equipment requisition; and equipment transport and restocking. *Major*-Standard with specialized equipment and/or microscopes and moderate body fluid/blood spillage. *Extensive*-Standard with extensive equipment (6 or more sets), or extensive radical surgery. Suite clean up is calculated by subtracting (-) the time the patient leaves the OR from the time of completion of the suite clean up times (x) number of nursing personnel.

Level	Weight	Ranges (minutes)
Standard	1	15 or less
Major	2	16-30
Extensive	4	31 or greater

Outpatient refers to day of surgery of same day surgery patients—those patients who are admitted, undergo surgical intervention, and are discharged in less than 24 hours. AM is for day of surgery admission patients—patients who are admitted prior to surgery. AM is intended to capture those patients admitted prior to surgery who will remain in the institution more than 24 hours following surgical intervention. Inpatient indicates a hospitalized patient. A surgical patient who is admitted prior to surgery, resides in a bed on the nursing unit, and who is expected to recover from surgical intervention within the institution for more than 24 hours. The admission status of the patient can be quickly circled to indicate whether the patient is outpatient, AM, or inpatient.

Indicator Definitions

Transport: Includes confirmation of patient's identity and determination of appropriate method for transport. Weights vary according to presence of patient support equipment (eg, monitors, suction, IVs) and location of unit.

Assessment: *Routine*-Includes routine history and physical, verification of procedure, review of patient record, and documentation. *Routine with monitor*-Includes routine assessment of a patient who has a monitor in place. *Extensive*-Includes routine assessment of a patient who has an extensive medical record requiring indepth history and physical. The patient *may* have monitor in place.

Medications: *PO, IM, IV fluids, add to IV, IV push*-Includes preparation, administration, evaluation, and charting. If more than one administration, multiply the number of administrations by the assigned weight. *Eye medications*-Includes instillation, monitoring, evaluation, and charting.

Safety/Comfort: *Secure belongings*-Includes assistance with undressing, identification, and placement of belongings. *Change position*-Includes general comfort measurers (eg, blanket, pillow, position change). If more than one comfort measure is provided, multiply the number by a weight of 1. *Assist with elimination*-Includes either assist to bathroom or use of bedpan/urinal. If done more than once, multiply by a weight of 1. *Emotional support*-Includes support given to patients/families that is *not* accompanied by other activities. If more than one occurrence, multiply by a weight of 1. *Constant monitoring*-Includes constant one to one ratio of care giver to patient.

Teaching: *Routine patient/family teaching*-Including content related to the surgical procedure *not* accompanied by other activities. *Discharge/Home care*-Routine teaching plus content related to discharge planning/home care.

Procedures: *Skin prep(limb)*-Includes preparation, skin shave, equipment disposal, and charting for preps performed on limbs or for minor skin surgeries. *Skin prep (trunk)*-Includes preparation, skin shave, equipment disposal, and charting for preps performed on the trunk or for removal of hardware. *Assist with A-line, breast measurement, fetal monitoring*-Includes procurement, preparation, assistance with procedure, disposal of equipment, and charting. *Epidural and axillary blocks*-Includes procurement, preparation, assistance with procedure, disposal of equipment, evaluation and charting.

Communication: *Charting, additional data*-Includes recording additional information, beyond that already associated with another activity (eg, lab/diagnostic reports). *Charting, extensive*-Includes ongoing progress notes and additional orders. *Collaboration*-Includes communicating/consulting with other professionals regarding changes in patient status or for situational problems.

Patient Condition: Includes patients with physical or mental disabilities, and/or the debilitated/frail elderly.

Suite preparation: Includes clock time multiplied by number of nursing personnel involved in setup for the procedure. Includes obtaining/positioning equipment and establishing/maintaining a sterile field.

Weights reflect total nursing time required.

Level	Weight	Ranges (minutes)
Minor	1	15 or less
Standard	2	16-30
Major	3	31-45
Extensive	6	46 or greater

Suite prep is calculated thus:

Time patient arrives in OR
-Time suite prep began
(minutes) × number of nursing personnel

Patient Preparation: Includes length of time required to prepare patient multiplied by number of nursing personnel involved. Includes reconfirming patient identity, surgical procedure, and consent; positioning; monitoring; preparing incision site; providing emotional support; establishing comfort/safety; assisting with induction; creating/maintaining sterile field; and monitoring the environment.

Weights reflect total nursing time required.

Level	Weight	Ranges (minutes)
Minor	2	30 or less
Standard	3	31-45
Major	5	46-75
Extensive I	7	76-105
Extensive II	14	106 or greater

Patient Prep is calculated thus:

Time incision made
-Time patient arrives in OR
(minutes) × number of nursing personnel

Surgical Procedure: Includes multiplying length of time from incision to when patient leaves OR by the number of nursing personnel involved. Assigned weights reflect total nursing time.

Level	Weight	Ranges (minutes)
Minor	4	60 or less
Standard	7	61-105
Major	12	106-180
Extensive I	20	181-300
Extensive II	33	301-495
Extensive III	58	496 or greater

Surgical Procedure is calculated thus:

Time patient leaves OR
-Time incision made
(minutes) × number of nursing personnel

Suite Clean Up: *Standard*-Includes all activities involved in decontamination of suite and the requisition of supplies and equipment. Includes equipment transport and restocking. Cases with minimal/standard equipment and minimal body fluid/blood spillage (eg, herniorrhaphy, biopsies). *Major*-Includes standard clean up on cases associated with specialized equipment and or microscopes and moderate body fluid/blood spillage (eg, cardiovascular procedures, laminectomy, abdominal procedures with double setup, mastectomy). *Extensive*-Includes standard clean up on cases requiring the use of extensive equipment (six or more sets) or extensive radical surgery.

Assigned weights reflect total nursing time.

Level	Weight	Ranges (minutes)
Standard	1	15 or less
Major	2	16-30
Extensive	4	31-60

Suite clean up is calculated thus:

Time suite clean up complete
-Time patient leaves OR
(minutes) × number of nursing personnel

CHAPTER 5
IMPLEMENTATION OF THE PATIENT CLASSIFICATION INSTRUMENT IN THE PREOPERATIVE SETTING

The preoperative phase, defined for the purposes of this instrument, begins with the transport of the patient to the preoperative/holding area or upon arrival of the patient in the preoperative/holding area and ends when the operating room nurse assumes responsibility for patient care. Preoperative indicators include transport, assessment, medications, comfort/safety, teaching, procedures, communication and patient condition. For the purposes of preoperative calculations, a unit of one is equal to three minutes of nursing time.

As discussed earlier, some facilities may find it necessary to alter the instrument. In that event, reliability and validity studies must be completed to ensure accuracy of the data collected. For instance, one alteration in the instrument might be the deletion of the skin prep activity from the tool because no skin preps are completed in the preoperative area contiguous to the operating room suite, but rather, are completed on the surgical unit prior to patient transfer to the holding area. In others, nursing staff are not responsible for assisting with epidural blocks because this is completed by the anesthesia team. In some facilities no preoperative holding area exists so preoperative patient classification would not be useful. Some facilities will require the addition of other indicators of nursing care such as removal of casts or the administration of enemas. The addition of these indicators would require reliability and validity studies.

The question of which staff should be included in tool calculations is often raised. The best rule of thumb to follow is that if the staff are a part of the surgical services payroll, they should be included in calculations for the tool. For instance, the time for anesthesiologists, nurse anesthetists, and surgeons is not calculated. Transporters, nursing assistants, volunteers, and housekeepers, who are not employed in the surgical services department, are not counted in calculations. Students, whether medical or nursing, also are not counted for the purposes of the study. Those individuals who are on orientation in the department should also not be calculated into the study until they are able to contribute to patient care as independent practitioners.

This section of the text will describe in detail the information contained in the preoperative section of the patient classification instrument and the preoperative acuity categories, and it will provide sample patient situations for scoring. The data shown was compiled from the timed sampling prior to reliability sampling.

Transport

Transport	
Floor/Unit	4
Floor/Unit with monitor	8
Intensive Care Unit	8
Floor/Unit special bed	12
Outpatient	0

Patient transport includes confirmation of the patient's identity and determination of appropriate methods of transport. Assigned weights vary according to the presence of patient support equipment and/or the location of the hospital surgical unit.

Patient transport was one of the most variable factors considered in the instrument because of the significant differences in facility layout and distances between the surgical units and the preoperative holding area. Patient transport timing began when the individual responsible for physically transporting the patient (ie, nursing assistant, orderly, LPN, RN) was notified that the patient should be obtained and transported to the surgical suite and/or the holding unit prior to surgical intervention. Notification of patient transport may be made verbally (eg, "please go to room 422 and pick up Mrs. Smith"), in writing (eg, handing the transporter a slip with the patient's name and room number), or in other ways. When patients transport themselves, as in the case of the ambulatory or AM admission patient, the timing begins when the nursing staff becomes responsible for the patient (eg, when the nursing assistant begins escort of the patient to the holding area). Timing of patient transport stops when the patient is moved to an assigned bed in the holding area (if he or she is an ambulatory or wheel chair patient) or when the stretcher/gurney is placed in the assigned preoperative space/bay. In essence, timing begins and ends based upon the nursing staff's assignment to a specific patient and their presence with the patient during transport.

Weights assigned to the patient transport indicator vary depending upon the location of the patient and the types of monitors/equipment that accompany the patient to the holding area. The ambulatory surgery patient who transports himself or herself to the holding area on the direction of the receptionist and who is unaccompanied by staff receives no score. In the research study, outpatient transport time was quite variable across sites. For instance, patients were escorted to the preoperative holding area by admission clerks or arrived unescorted; if nursing personnel were involved, mean times ranged from one minute to 8.54 minutes, depending upon the distance of the waiting area from the holding area.

Patients who are transported by the staff from the surgical floor/unit to the surgical suite receive a basic score of 4. Other scores are increased based upon the addition of monitors, special beds, and transport from an intensive care area, which usually indicates additional staff. During timing studies conducted to validate the instrument, the mean time necessary to transport patients from a hospital unit to the preoperative holding area was 12.58 minutes (SD=6.05). Further review of the transport data found the average time of transport was increased by a factor of two when patients were electronically monitored, or were receiving two or three intravenous fluids and/or oxygen. When a special bed was used to transport the patient, nursing time was increased by a factor of 3. Weights of 8 and 12 were thus assigned to these variations in transport time. For example, a patient transported from the surgical unit to the preoperative holding area by the nursing assistant would receive a score of 4. A patient with three IV's and portable oxygen transported from the Intensive Care Unit by an RN would receive a score of 8. Those patients transported by special flotation or orthopedic beds would receive a score of 12.

When considering assigned units for the transport indicator, it well be helpful to remember that each unit in the preoperative section of the tool is equal to three minutes of nursing time. Therefore, transport from the floor/unit to the holding area has a unit score of four and is equal to approximately 12 minutes of nursing time. Transport from the floor/unit with a monitor in place has a unit of eight and thus equates to approximately 24 minutes. The same is true of transport from the intensive care unit. Transport from the floor/unit in a special bed is a unit of 12 and can be accomplished in approximately 36 minutes. The increasing numbers of nursing personnel required to transport the patient are included in the unit calculations. Therefore, the unit of eight for floor/unit with monitor, accounts for two transporters while the floor/unit with a score of four accounts for only one transporter.

Patient transport is one of the most variable factors considered in the instrument. Each institution should consider conducting timing studies to validate the weights assigned as a result of the study.

ASSESSMENT

Assessment	
Routine	2
Routine with monitor	3
Extensive	4

Preoperative patient assessment is categorized as routine, routine with monitor, and extensive. Routine patient assessment includes completion of a basic health history and physical assessment, verification of the surgical procedure to be performed, review of the patient's record, and documentation of observations/data. Timing of nursing assessment activities begins when the nurse approached the patient's bed and ends when the charting is completed at either the bedside or at a desk. The timing for patient assessment also includes the retrieval of routine lab data either in writing or orally.

Preoperative assessment data were divided into groups based on the distribution of scores. Although a majority of assessments (88%) were completed in 10 minutes or less, (mean = 5.27 minutes), the remaining 12% of assessments ranged from 10 to 30 minutes with a mean of 13.22 minutes. The mean for all assessments was 5.83 minutes. Longer assessments were usually associated with critically ill patients, patients who had intermittent monitoring, or patients who required a lengthy chart review. A weight of 2 was assigned to routine assessments.

Routine assessment with monitor includes the same activities identified for routine assessment, but in this instance, the patient has an electronic monitor in place. These monitors may be fetal monitors, heart monitors, or other monitoring equipment that require only periodic ongoing assessment and do not require constant attention. Because more nursing time is required to care for patients with monitors in place, the score for routine assessment with monitor is 3. Utilizing three minutes equal to one unit, the time to complete routine assessment with monitor is approximately nine minutes.

Extensive assessment involves the same activities identified for routine assessment, but the patient has a more extensive medical record and requires and in-depth history/physical assessment due to the extent of the illness or condition. Patients who require extensive assessments may or may not have an electronic monitor in place. As a result of the additional nursing time required for assessment of the critically ill patient, a score of 4 was assigned.

An example of routine assessment would be the healthy adult admitted for breast augmentation. Routine laboratory work would be obtained and a basic assessment completed. The assessment would be termed routine with monitor if the patient scheduled for the breast augmentation had a history of cardiac arrhythmia and was placed on a cardiac monitor for observation only. An extensive assessment would include the trauma patient admitted directly from the Emergency Room to the preoperative holding area. Based on the scarcity of information provided about the patient, an extensive nursing assessment and access to laboratory and radiology information would be necessary.

MEDICATIONS

Medications			
IM injection	1 ×	___	= ___
Add to IV bag	1 ×	___	= ___
IV fluid administration	2 ×	___	= ___
IV meds (push)	2 ×	___	= ___
Eye meds	4		
			Subtotal

The third category of indicators is medications and includes the administration of intravenous fluids. Medications administered by mouth, intramuscularly, and through intravenous fluids are calculated include preparation, administration, evaluation of the outcomes of medication administration, and charting. If more than one medication or IV fluid is administered, the number of medications or IV fluids given is multiplied by the assigned weights to obtain a score.

The timing of IV and medication administration begins with procurement of the IV or medication (eg, taking it from the shelf) and is concluded at the completion of charting. It was necessary in timing the IV preparation to note when the RN started and stopped some activities associated with IV and medication administration. For instance, the preparation and final insertion of the IV may not be one single process. The RN may obtain the IV fluids, assemble the bag, label the solution with the patient's name and hang the bag. The work may then be interrupted because the patient is not available for insertion of the line. The bag is then placed at an appropriate spot to be obtained later when the actual insertion and infusion of the solution will occur. Nursing time would not be calculated when the IV fluid bag was ready for infusion but was not yet being infused.

The study found that the average time to administer medications varied by route of administration. Intramuscular injections and the addition of a medication to an IV bag averaged 3.20 minutes; intravenous fluid infusion and IV medication direct injection (ie, IV push) increased the time factor by two. Therefore, the process of preparing and administering an IM injection received a score of 1. The addition of a medication to an already hanging IV solution also is scored as 1. However, if several medications are added to the solution, the number added should be multiplied by 1 to obtain the actual score. For instance, Mrs. Smith has a solution of dextrose and water hanging. The order is to add 20 meg. of KCL and 1 GM of Ampicillin. The resultant score for that nursing activity would be 2 (ie, 2 medications [KCL and Ampicillin] times the factor of 1) and would have taken approximately six minutes to accomplish (ie, 3 minutes, times the factor of 2).

The preparation and administration of IV fluids and IV medications delivered by IV injections receives a score of 2 and is multiplied by the number of IV fluids and IV medications prepared and administered. During the study, IV fluid administration (including setup) mean time was 6.44 minutes and therefore received a weight of two in light of comparison with the mean time of 3.2 minutes to prepare and administer an IM injection or add a medication to in infusing fluid line.

The instillation of eye medication received a weight of 4 and averaged 4.21 minutes in the study. A weight of 4 was calculated as the result of two units representing the average time required for multiple installations (mean=3.87 minutes) and two units representing the time the RN spends evaluating the effectiveness of the medication.

COMFORT/SAFETY

Comfort/Safety	
Secure belongings	1
Help change position	1 × ____ = ____
Assist with elimination	1 × ____ = ____
Emotional support (patient/family)	1 × ____ = ____
Constant monitoring	8
	Subtotal

Several activities were grouped under the category of comfort/safety measures. These activities include: secure patient belongings, change patient position, assist patient with elimination (ambulatory or bedpan), provide emotional support (includes patient and family) and constant monitoring. Mean times for securing belongings and comfort measures were 0.94 and 0.96 minutes respectively; assisting with elimination was 2.87 minutes; and providing emotional support was 2.92 minutes. Each of these activities received a weight of 1. Patients requiring constant monitoring received a score of 8; this assignment was a judgment based upon the sample clock time mean in the preoperative holding area (45.50 minutes) minus the mean preoperative nursing time (15.14 minutes).

The timing for secure belongings included assistance with undressing and identification and placement of belongings. Patients who arrive in the preoperative holding area fully clothed require the assistance of nursing personnel in undressing, identifying, and securing belongings. Elderly patients who arrive in the preoperative holding area may need assistance in both undressing and securing belongings while a healthy young patient may require only direction as to where to go to change clothes and assistance in securing the belongings in a safe area while the surgery is being performed. A score of 1 was assigned to the activity "secure belongings." In some instances no score will be given to the patient who arrives in the preoperative holding area already suitably dressed for surgery.

The help change position indicator includes general comfort measures such as getting extra blankets, and/or pillows, and/or assisting with position changes. This comfort measure is designed to assist the patient in feeling comfortable in the preoperative area. In instances where patients remain in the preoperative holding area for a long time, several measures may be taken to assist with positioning. In that event, the factor of 1 would be multiplied by the number of occurrences (eg, assisting the patient in severe pain with positioning may occur several times during their preoperative holding area stay).

Assist with elimination includes either assistance to the bathroom or use of the bedpan or urinal. This activity is given a score of one. However, it should be noted that extended stays in the preoperative holding area again may result in the need to multiply the factor 1 by the number of times the patient is assisted with elimination. For instance, in some facilities, the patient is admitted to the preoperative holding area for enema administration. These patients may require assistance to the bathroom on several occasions. The number of times that nursing personnel assist the patient would be multiplied by the factor 1.

Another comfort/safety measure considered important in development of the tool was emotional support. This was defined to include emotional support given to the patient, family member(s), and/or significant others. It was designed to measure emotional support provided in the absence of other activities. For instance, if the nursing personnel approach the patient to start an IV and in the process offer the patient emotional support regarding his or her surgery, then no score would be calculated for emotional support but the factor 2 would be identified for the IV fluid administration. If, however, the nurse attends to the emotional support of the patient when no other activity accompanies it, then the score would be given as 1. Another example would be assistance with an elderly patient. The nurse may approach the patient to give an intramuscular injection and stay with the patient for a few moments to provide a supportive measure (eg, touching). No additional score would be given for that activity. If however, the nurse returns to the bedside on additional occasions following the injection to address the emotional needs of the family by providing comfort that would be scored as the factor 1 times the number of supportive activity occurrences.

The constant monitoring indicator is included to account for the patient who requires constant one-to-one care. It is scored as an 8 because of the intensity of nursing care required to care for the patient. Instances of constant monitoring would be the multiple trauma patient who requires constant attention to the cardiac monitor prior to movement to the operating room. It should be recognized that there may be several personnel attending to the emergency patient. In that event, the scores would be calculated for each activity, regardless of the number of personnel. One patient in critical condition may require the attention of three nursing personnel simultaneously conducting assessment, administering IV fluids and medications and monitoring cardiac status. In that event, all activities would be calculated regardless of the number of personnel involved in the care.

TEACHING

Teaching	
Routine re: surgery (patient or family)	1
Discharge/Home care (patient or family)	2
	Subtotal

Two levels of teaching were identified in the study. The majority (71%) of patient and/or family teaching activities addressed concerns regarding surgery (routine) and were 3.5 minutes or less. The calculation of routine surgery teaching only should be included if the content is related to the immediate surgical experience and is not done in conjunction with any other activity. A weight of 1 was assigned to this activity.

Longer teaching episodes involved same day surgery patients and/or their families and included postoperative discharge planning. These sessions ranged from 4.50 to 7.00 minutes. This activity only should be included if the content of the teaching is related to issues beyond the immediate surgical procedure, such as discharge planning and/or home care instructions. A weight of 2 was assigned to discharge planning teaching.

It should be noted that these teaching activities should only be added to the cumulative score if the teaching episodes are not accompanied by other activities. If the nursing personnel are engaged in teaching the patient at the same time as they are administering medications or providing comfort, the scores should only reflect the more intense activity and not both activities.

An example of routine surgical teaching would be teaching conducted for the hysterectomy patient. Routine teaching methods and patient pamphlets would be reviewed and discussed. Extensive teaching would include teaching conducted for the patient scheduled for laparoscopic cholecystectomy on an ambulatory basis. The time required to adequately teach the patient postoperative care could be much longer because of the need for the patient to control their own care upon discharge.

PROCEDURES

Procedures	
Skin prep: (limb)	1
Skin prep: (trunk)	2
Assist A-line	3
Assist breast measurement	3
Fetal monitoring	5
Epidural blocks	6
Axillary blocks	4
	Subtotal

Several types of procedures were observed when the nurse assisted the physician. With the exception of skin preparation and/or shave, these procedures involved arterial line placement, breast measurement, fetal monitor placement, and epidural and axillary blocks. Although relatively few timed observations were obtained on these procedures, the amount of nursing time involved in these activities made it necessary to include these procedures on the instrument's inventory.

Mean nursing time to prepare incision sites was 5.70 minutes; however it was observed that in general, limb preparation and preparation of sites in which surgical procedures involved removal of benign lesion (eg, Nevi), the mean time was 3.49 minutes. When surgery involved the trunk or removal of hardware, the mean time increased to 5.80 minutes. Based on these findings, weights of 1 and 2 were assigned depending on the incision site. Skin preparation/shave activities were timed to include preparation, shave, disposal of equipment, and charting. The limb preparation category is used if the skin preparation includes a limb or other minor skin area. The trunk preparation activity, scored as 2, includes the skin prep of a patient's trunk or skin prep for the removal of hardware. For instance, a patient shaved and prepared for an open heart procedure would be scored as a 2 while a patient who was shaved and prepped for the removal of a nevus would receive a score of 1.

Assistance provided to physicians during arterial line placements (n = 3) and breast measurement (n = 4) each received weights of 3. Fetal monitor placement (n = 2) was assigned a weight of 5. These timing activities include the procurement, preparation, assistance with the procedure, disposal of equipment, and charting as a part of the timing studies.

Preoperative activities also included assistance with epidural and axillary blocks. Both of these activities were timed, and average weights were assigned. Epidural blocks received a weight of 6 as a result of a mean time of 17.73 minutes and axillary blocks were assigned a weight of 4, with a mean time of 12.83 minutes. These timings reflect the procurement, preparation, assistance with the procedure, disposal of the equipment, charting, and evaluation of the effectiveness of the block.

COMMUNICATION

Communication	
Charting-add data	1
-extensive	2
Collaboration	1
	Subtotal

Communication included both written documentation on patient records and phone calls for the purpose of obtaining more information such as laboratory or radiology reports. Professional collaboration was included under communication, but was viewed as a separate activity involving oral interchange with other health professionals regarding a change in patient status or situational problems.

The average time for written documentation (eg, charting) was 4.56 minutes, however two time levels were identified. The first level reflected recording of additional data such as laboratory reports. The mean time for this activity was 2.31 minutes, but 19.4% of charting episodes included more extensive documentation and averaged 6.80 minutes. Weights of 1 and 2 were assigned to reflect these two mean values. Charting of additional data includes the recording of additional information, such as laboratory or other diagnostic reports. It includes the time when the nurse determines the additional information is needed and accesses that information from another department either orally or in writing. Extensive charting includes the ongoing progress notes and additional orders based on the patient's status. An example of routine charting would be included in the documentation for a female patient who is undergoing laparoscopic exam for which a pregnancy test is required according to institutional policy. Extensive charting would include the patient who upon assessment is determined to be at risk for malignant hyperthermia. The nurse would determine what additional laboratory tests should be obtained prior to surgery.

Professional collaboration received a weight of 1, based on a mean of 1.72 minutes. Collaboration involves communicating or consulting with other nursing or health professionals regarding changes in patient status or situational problems. An example would be the patient who is at risk for developing malignant hyperthermia. The collaboration would occur among the health care providers assigned to the care of the patient (eg, anesthesia personnel, nursing personnel, pharmacy, and the surgeon).

PATIENT CONDITION

Patient Condition	
Disability (blind, deaf, communication barrier, cognitive, foreign lang)	2

Preoperative data were reviewed on patients who were identified by the data collectors' written comments as disabled or being frail elderly, or debilitated, and the indicator "patient condition" was added to the tool. Fifteen patients were identified who met these characteristics. Patient disabilities included blindness (n = 2); mobility (n = 3); mental disorientation/retardation (n = 3); and the frail elderly or debilitated patient (n = 7). The mean preoperative time (excluding patient transport time) was compared to the sample mean (ie, 21.73 to 15.50 minutes) and an equivalent weight of 2 was assigned to patient condition as a result.

Those patients who might require additional attention as a result of their condition include patients who have problems with mobility, mental retardation, mental disorientation, blindness, deafness, cognitive dissonance, communication barriers such as foreign language or debility. An example of a patient who is included in this category would be the mentally retarded patient who is scheduled for bilateral myringotomy.

PREOPERATIVE PATIENT ACUITY CATEGORIES

Preoperative Acuity Categories
Total Pre op score_____
Circle one:
7 or less   Category I
8 to 10   Category II
11 +   Category III

To identify patient acuity categories for the preoperative period, total sample data were examined. The distribution of patient scores (including patient transport time) revealed the following information: 44% of the sample scores were 21 minutes or less (Level 1); 32% of the scores were between 21.1 and 30.09 minutes (Level II); the remaining 24% of scores were above 45 minutes. The mean times for these three levels were: Level I, 13.64 minutes; Level II, 24.55 minutes; and Level III, 40.09 minutes. A decision was made to accept these levels as acuity categories. Equivalent units based on 3.0 minutes or less per unit were assigned to reflect acuity time intervals associated with these categories: Category I was equivalent to 7 units or less; Category II, 8 to 10 units; and Category III, 11 or more units. Thus, a patient with an acuity Category I requires up to 21 minutes of total nursing care. Category II requires 24 to 30 minutes of nursing care, and Category III requires 33 or more minutes of nursing care. Preoperative Acuity Categories and their resultant weights and ranges are summarized as follows:

Level	Weights (units)	Ranges (minutes)
Category I	7 or less	21
Category II	8-10	24-30
Category III	11 or more	33 or greater

The acuity category is determined by adding the scores circled or calculated for the eight preoperative indicators. The total score of 7 or less equals an acuity category of I (21 minutes of nursing care or less); a total score 8 to 10 would indicate an acuity category of II (24 to 30 minutes of nursing care); and a total score of 11 or more would indicate an acuity category of III (33 minutes or more of nursing care).

Samples of Preoperative Timing Activities

This section of the preoperative chapter will demonstrate implementation of the instrument using written patient simulation exercises. Two preoperative simulations are presented. Readers are encouraged to review the definitions for preoperative indicators of care (see page 16) and complete the preoperative section of the AORN Patient Classification Instrument sample on the following page. Compute the total preoperative score and assign the appropriate acuity category.

PATIENT SIMULATION #1

Otto Carns, age 87, is accompanied from home by his daughter to the holding area of the hospital operating room at 7:30 a.m. He is scheduled for removal of a cataract and insertion of an intraocular lens in his right eye at 9:45 a.m. He had the same procedure done on his left eye about 9 months ago, but has suffered several small strokes in the meantime and is currently somewhat agitated, forgetful, and very hard of hearing.

The nurse and Mr. Carns' daughter, Lorraine, assist him to undress and put on the surgical gown. He finds it very difficult to lie down on the stretcher due to emphysema and arthritis in his spine. The nurse adjusts the backrest of the stretcher and carefully positions two extra pillows before he says he is comfortable. She completes her intake assessment which entails a brief history.

The nurse begins the administration of mydriatic-cycloplegic and prophylactic antibiotic eye drops prescribed by Mr. Carns' surgeon. These are scheduled over one hour with four specific installations. Mr. Carns has difficulty lying still and keeping his eye open during the installations and attempts to push the nurse's hands away. His

AORN PATIENT CLASSIFICATION
Preoperative

Admission Status:
Outpatient, AM, Inpatient
Procedure: _____

Transport

Floor/Unit	4
Floor/Unit with monitor	8
Intensive Care unit	8
Floor/Unit special bed	12
Outpatient	0

Assessment

Routine	2
Routine with monitor	3
Extensive	4

Medications

IM injection	1 × ___ =
Add to IV bag	1 × ___ =
IV fluid administration	2 × ___ =
IV meds (push)	2 × ___ =
Eye meds	4
	Subtotal

Comfort/Safety

Secure belongings	1 × ___ =
Help change position	1 × ___ =
Assist with elimination	1 × ___ =
Emotional support (patient/family)	1 × ___ =
Constant monitoring	8
	Subtotal

Teaching

Routine re: surgery (patient or family)	1
Discharge/Home care (patient or family)	2
	Subtotal

Procedures

Skin prep: (limb)	1
Skin prep: (trunk)	2
Assist A-line	3
Assist breast measurement	3
Fetal monitoring	5
Epidural blocks	6
Axillary blocks	4
	Subtotal

Communication

Charting-add data	1
-extensive	2
Collaboration	1
	Subtotal

Patient Condition

Disability (blind, deaf, communication barrier, cognitive, foreign lang)	2

Preoperative Acuity Categories

Total Pre op score _____
Circle one:
7 or less	Category I
8 to 10	Category II
11 +	Category III

Admission Status: Circle type of patient outpatient, (AM) patient admitted day of surgery, or inpatient.

Transport: Identification of patient, determination of appropriate method of transport, and transport accomplished. Varies according to presence of patient support equipment (monitors, suctions, IV's) and location of hospital unit.

Assessment: *Routine*-History and physical, verification of procedure, review of patient record and documentation. *Routine with monitor*-Routine assessment/monitor in place. *Extensive*-Routine assessment/extensive may have monitor.

Medications: *PO, IM, IV fluids, add to IV, IV push*-Includes preparation, administration, evaluation, and charting. If more than one, multiply number by assigned weight. *Eye medications*-Includes instillation, monitoring, evaluation, and charting.

Comfort/Safety: *Secure belongings*-Assistance with undressing, identification and placement of belongings. *Help change position*-General comfort measurers (blanket, pillow, position change). Multiply by weight of 1. *Assist with elimination*-Assist to bathroom or use of bedpan/urinal. Multiply by weight of 1. *Emotional support*-Support given not accompanied by other activities. Multiply by weight of 1. *Constant monitoring*-Constant one-to-one ratio of care.

Teaching: *Routine-* Patient/family teaching including content related to surgical procedure not accompanied by other activities. *Discharge/Home Care*-Routine plus content related to discharge planning/home care.

Procedures: *Skin prep*-Preparation, skin shave, equipment disposal, and charting for preps performed on limbs/trunks. *Assist with A-line, breast measurement, fetal monitoring*-Procurement, preparation, assistance with procedure, disposal of equipment, and charting. *Epidural and axillary blocks*-Procurement, preparation, assistance with procedure, disposal of equipment, evaluation, and charting.

Communication: *Charting, additional data*-Recording additional information, beyond that associated with other activities. *Charting, extensive*-Ongoing progress notes, and additional orders. *Collaboration*-Communicating/consulting with others regarding changes in patient status/situational problems.

Patient Condition: Patients with physical or mental disability, communication barrier, and/or debilitated/frail elderly.

Version 9
4/92

daughter stays beside him and offers quieting reassurnaces.

At 9.20 a.m., Mr. Carns' surgeon, Dr. Glass, stops by and visits with the patient and his daughter. He reviews the major points of the surgery that have been discussed in the office and reaffirms that Mr. Carns will be able to return home this afternoon. At 9:30 Mr. Carns is taken to the operating room by the perioperative nurse.

In determining the acuity category for Mr. Carns, it becomes evident that the score for patient transport is 0 since no nursing personnel were responsible for transporting the patient to the preoperative holding area. The assessment entailed a brief history and would be routine with a score of 2. Mr. Carns received eye drops and thus receives a score of 4. The nurse and the daughter assisted the patient in undressing and the score for secure belongings is 1. The nurse provided comfort by positioning Mr. Carns with two pillows. That results in a score of 1 for helps change position. The subtotal score for comfort/safety is 2. Mr. Carns surgeon visited with the patient and no note was made of teaching provided to the patient. Therefore, the score in that category is 0. No procedures were performed for Mr. Carns and no additional charting was completed. Therefore, the scores for both procedures and communication are 0. As a result of Mr. Carns difficulty in hearing, he receives a score of 2 for patient condition. The total score for Mr. Carns is 10.

Transport	0
Assessment	2
Medications	4
Comfort/Safety	2
Teaching	0
Procedures	0
Communications	0
Patient condition	2
Total Score	10

Patient preoperative score of 10 equals an Acuity Category rating of II.

AORN PATIENT CLASSIFICATION
Preoperative

Admission Status: (Outpatient) AM, Inpatient
Procedure: Cataract extraction w/IOL inserted

Transport
Floor/Unit	4
Floor/Unit with monitor	8
Intensive Care unit	8
Floor/Unit special bed	12
Outpatient	(0)

Assessment
Routine	(2)
Routine with monitor	3
Extensive	4

Medications
IM injection	1 × ___ =	
Add to IV bag	1 × ___ =	
IV fluid administration	2 × ___ =	
IV meds (push)	2 × ___ =	
Eye meds	(4)	
	Subtotal	4

Comfort/Safety
Secure belongings	(1) × ___ =	
Help change position	1 × 1 =	1
Assist with elimination	1 × ___ =	
Emotional support (patient/family)	1 × ___ =	
Constant monitoring	8	
	Subtotal	2

Teaching
Routine re: surgery (patient or family)	1
Discharge/Home care (patient or family)	2
Subtotal	0

Procedures
Skin prep: (limb)	1
Skin prep: (trunk)	2
Assist A-line	3
Assist breast measurement	3
Fetal monitoring	5
Epidural blocks	6
Axillary blocks	4
Subtotal	0

Communication
Charting-add data	1
-extensive	2
Collaboration	1
Subtotal	0

Patient Condition
Disability (blind, deaf, communication barrier, cognitive, foreign lang)	(2)

Preoperative Acuity Categories
Total Pre op score __10__
Circle one:
- 7 or less — Category I
- (8 to 10) — (Category II)
- 11 + — Category III

Admission Status: Circle type of patient outpatient, (AM) patient admitted day of surgery, or inpatient.

Transport: Identification of patient, determination of appropriate method of transport, and transport accomplished. Varies according to presence of patient support equipment (monitors, suctions, IV's) and location of hospital unit.

Assessment: *Routine*-History and physical, verification of procedure, review of patient record and documentation. *Routine with monitor*-Routine assessment/monitor in place. *Extensive*-Routine assessment/extensive may have monitor.

Medications: *PO, IM, IV fluids, add to IV, IV push*-. Includes preparation, administration, evaluation, and charting. If more than one, multiply number by assigned weight. *Eye medications*-Includes instillation, monitoring, evaluation, and charting.

Comfort/Safety: *Secure belongings*-Assistance with undressing, identification and placement of belongings. *Help change position*-General comfort measurers (blanket, pillow, position change). Multiply by weight of 1. *Assist with elimination*-Assist to bathroom or use of bedpan/urinal. Multiply by weight of 1. *Emotional support*-Support given not accompanied by other activities. Multiply by weight of 1. *Constant monitoring*-Constant one-to-one ratio of care.

Teaching: *Routine*-Patient/family teaching including content related to surgical procedure not accompanied by other activities. *Discharge/Home Care*-Routine plus content related to discharge planning/home care.

Procedures: *Skin prep*-Preparation, skin shave, equipment disposal, and charting for preps performed on limbs/trunks. *Assist with A-line, breast measurement, fetal monitoring*-Procurement, preparation, assistance with procedure, disposal of equipment, and charting. *Epidural and axillary blocks*-Procurement, preparation, assistance with procedure, disposal of equipment, evaluation, and charting.

Communication: *Charting, additional data*-Recording additional information, beyond that associated with other activities. *Charting, extensive*-Ongoing progress notes, and additional orders. *Collaboration*-Communicating/consulting with others regarding changes in patient status/situational problems.

Patient Condition: Patients with physical or mental disability, communication barrier, and/or debilitated/frail elderly.

Version 9
4/92

PATIENT SIMULATION #2

Carol Smith, age 64, is a patient in CCU and is scheduled for triple bypass surgery at 10 a.m. The RN and orderly from the holding area transport her to the holding area by stretcher. Ms. Smith was admitted to the hospital two days ago after her husband brought her to the Emergency Room when she experienced an acute coronary occlusion at home. According to her chart and the oral history taken by the holding area nurse, Ms. Smith stabilized rather quickly following her admission. Although she is still being continuously monitored, she is considered an excellent candidate for this surgery. Her general health is good.

The holding area nurse performs a venipuncture and hangs a bag of Ringer's lactate. Ms. Smith's family physician and the cardiac surgeon, Dr. Valentine, visit with Ms. Smith and her husband. Dr. Valentine requests the nurse's assistance in starting an arterial line.

Ms. Smith becomes very frightened and begins to cry after her surgeon leaves the holding area. The nurse stands calmly beside her stretcher, holds her hand, and listens as she explains that this is her first time to have surgery and, even though she has faith in her doctors, she is afraid. The nurse offers positive support and reassurance. Ms. Smith is transported to the OR at 9:30 a.m.

AORN PATIENT CLASSIFICATION
Preoperative

Admission Status:
Outpatient, AM, Inpatient
Procedure: _____

Transport

Floor/Unit	4
Floor/Unit with monitor	8
Intensive Care unit	8
Floor/Unit special bed	12
Outpatient	0

Assessment

Routine	2
Routine with monitor	3
Extensive	4

Medications

IM injection	1 × ____	=
Add to IV bag	1 × ____	=
IV fluid administration	2 × ____	=
IV meds (push)	2 × ____	=
Eye meds	4	
	Subtotal	

Comfort/Safety

Secure belongings	1 × ____	=
Help change position	1 × ____	=
Assist with elimination	1 × ____	=
Emotional support (patient/family)	1 × ____	=
Constant monitoring	8	
	Subtotal	

Teaching

Routine re: surgery (patient or family)	1
Discharge/Home care (patient or family)	2
Subtotal	

Procedures

Skin prep: (limb)	1
Skin prep: (trunk)	2
Assist A-line	3
Assist breast measurement	3
Fetal monitoring	5
Epidural blocks	6
Axillary blocks	4
Subtotal	

Communication

Charting-add data	1
-extensive	2
Collaboration	1
Subtotal	

Patient Condition

Disability (blind, deaf, communication barrier, cognitive, foreign lang)	2

Preoperative Acuity Categories

Total Pre op score _____
Circle one:

7 or less	Category I
8 to 10	Category II
11 +	Category III

Admission Status: Circle type of patient outpatient, (AM) patient admitted day of surgery, or inpatient.

Transport: Identification of patient, determination of appropriate method of transport, and transport accomplished. Varies according to presence of patient support equipment (monitors, suctions, IV's) and location of hospital unit.

Assessment: *Routine*-History and physical, verification of procedure, review of patient record and documentation. *Routine with monitor*-Routine assessment/monitor in place. *Extensive*-Routine assessment/extensive may have monitor.

Medications: *PO, IM, IV fluids, add to IV, IV push*-Includes preparation, administration, evaluation, and charting. If more than one, multiply number by assigned weight. *Eye medications*-Includes instillation, monitoring, evaluation, and charting.

Comfort/Safety: *Secure belongings*-Assistance with undressing, identification and placement of belongings. *Help change position*-General comfort measurers (blanket, pillow, position change). Multiply by weight of 1. *Assist with elimination*- Assist to bathroom or use of bedpan/urinal. Multiply by weight of 1. *Emotional support*-Support given not accompanied by other activities. Multiply by weight of 1. *Constant monitoring*-Constant one-to-one ratio of care.

Teaching: *Routine*-Patient/family teaching including content related to surgical procedure not accompanied by other activities. *Discharge/Home Care*-Routine plus content related to discharge planning/home care.

Procedures: *Skin prep*-Preparation, skin shave, equipment disposal, and charting for preps performed on limbs/trunks. *Assist with A-line, breast measurement, fetal monitoring*-Procurement, preparation, assistance with procedure, disposal of equipment, and charting. *Epidural and axillary blocks*-Procurement, preparation, assistance with procedure, disposal of equipment, evaluation, and charting.

Communication: *Charting, additional data*-Recording additional information, beyond that associated with other activities. *Charting, extensive*-Ongoing progress notes, and additional orders. *Collaboration*-Communicating/consulting with others regarding changes in patient status/situational problems.

Patient Condition: Patients with physical or mental disability, communication barrier, and/or debilitated/frail elderly.

Version 9
4/92

In determining the Acuity Category for Ms. Smith, the following information is useful. Ms. Smith is transported to the preoperative holding area from the CCU, which indicates a score of 8. A routine assessment is completed, and the patient has a heart monitor in place. The score for assessment is 3. The IV is started and therefore a score of 2 is assigned to the medications category. The nurse provided emotional support, not in conjunction with any other activity for Ms. Smith, and the score for comfort/safety is 1. No teaching was given to Ms. Smith at this time, no additional charting was completed, and the patient condition did not indicate any disabilities. Thus, teaching and communication and patient condition receive scores of 0. The nurse assisted Dr. Valentine with the insertion of an arterial line and the score for procedures is 3. The total patient preoperative score is 17.

Transport	8
Assessment	3
Medications	2
Comfort/Safety	1
Teaching	0
Procedures	3
Communications	0
Patient Condition	0
Total Score	17

Patient preoperative score of 17 equals an Acuity Category rating of III.

AORN PATIENT CLASSIFICATION
Preoperative

Admission Status: Outpatient, AM, (Inpatient) [circled]
Procedure: Coronary Artery Bypass graft - 3

Transport
Floor/Unit	4
Floor/Unit with monitor	8
Intensive Care unit	(8) [circled]
Floor/Unit special bed	12
Outpatient	0

Assessment
Routine	2
Routine with monitor	(3) [circled]
Extensive	4

Medications
IM injection	1 × ___ =	
Add to IV bag	1 × ___ =	
IV fluid administration	2 × 1 =	2
IV meds (push)	2 × ___ =	
Eye meds	4	
	Subtotal	2

Comfort/Safety
Secure belongings	1 × ___ =	
Help change position	1 × ___ =	
Assist with elimination	1 × ___ =	
Emotional support (patient/family)	1 × 1 =	1
Constant monitoring	8	
	Subtotal	1

Teaching
Routine re: surgery (patient or family)	1
Discharge/Home care (patient or family)	2
Subtotal	0

Procedures
Skin prep: (limb)	1
Skin prep: (trunk)	2
Assist A-line	(3) [circled]
Assist breast measurement	3
Fetal monitoring	5
Epidural blocks	6
Axillary blocks	4
Subtotal	3

Communication
Charting-add data	1
-extensive	2
Collaboration	1
Subtotal	0

Patient Condition
Disability (blind, deaf, communication barrier, cognitive, foreign lang)	2
	0

Preoperative Acuity Categories
Total Pre op score: 17
Circle one:
- 7 or less — Category I
- 8 to 10 — Category II
- (11+) — Category III [circled]

Admission Status: Circle type of patient outpatient, (AM) patient admitted day of surgery, or inpatient.

Transport: Identification of patient, determination of appropriate method of transport, and transport accomplished. Varies according to presence of patient support equipment (monitors, suctions, IV's) and location of hospital unit.

Assessment: *Routine*-History and physical, verification of procedure, review of patient record and documentation. *Routine with monitor*-Routine assessment/monitor in place. *Extensive*-Routine assessment/extensive may have monitor.

Medications: *PO, IM, IV fluids, add to IV, IV push*-Includes preparation, administration, evaluation, and charting. If more than one, multiply number by assigned weight. *Eye medications*-Includes instillation, monitoring, evaluation, and charting.

Comfort/Safety: *Secure belongings*-Assistance with undressing, identification and placement of belongings. *Help change position*-General comfort measurers (blanket, pillow, position change). Multiply by weight of 1. *Assist with elimination*-Assist to bathroom or use of bedpan/urinal. Multiply by weight of 1. *Emotional support*-Support given not accompanied by other activities. Multiply by weight of 1. *Constant monitoring*- Constant one-to-one ratio of care.

Teaching: *Routine*-Patient/family teaching including content related to surgical procedure not accompanied by other activities. *Discharge/Home Care*- Routine plus content related to discharge planning/home care.

Procedures: *Skin prep*-Preparation, skin shave, equipment disposal, and charting for preps performed on limbs/trunks. *Assist with A-line, breast measurement, fetal monitoring*-Procurement, preparation, assistance with procedure, disposal of equipment, and charting. *Epidural and axillary blocks*-Procurement, preparation, assistance with procedure, disposal of equipment, evaluation, and charting.

Communication: *Charting, additional data*-Recording additional information, beyond that associated with other activities. *Charting, extensive*-Ongoing progress notes, and additional orders. *Collaboration*-Communicating/consulting with others regarding changes in patient status/situational problems.

Patient Condition: Patients with physical or mental disability, communication barrier, and/or debilitated/frail elderly.

Version 9
4/92

CHAPTER 6

IMPLEMENTATION OF THE PATIENT CLASSIFICATION INSTRUMENT IN THE INTRAOPERATIVE SETTING

The intraoperative phase of the perioperative period is probably the one most familiar to perioperative nurses. It is operationally defined for the purposes of this study as beginning when the operating room nurse assumes responsibility for the patient and ends when the suite clean up is completed. Unlike the preoperative phase during which the acuity categories are determined by the procedures and activities the nursing personnel perform for the patient, the intraoperative indicators are based on time increments. This is due to the assumption that the intraoperative period, regardless of the number of procedures performed for each patient, is a factor of the number of nursing personnel involved in the care of the patient for specified periods of time.

The intraoperative nursing activities were categorized into four major areas or indicators of care: suite preparation, patient preparation, surgical procedure, and suite clean up. Each indicator was divided into incremental time levels determined by the indicator's distribution of times.

Intraoperative acuity categories were established based on the distribution of the total intraoperative times (ie, sum of times obtained on the four indicators). Intra-indicator scales and intraoperative acuity categories were originally based on 1 unit for each 20 minutes. However, review of the empirical means for each level across indicators found that a 15 minute unit denoted more accurately the weight average for the levels.

Determining nursing time is sometimes a confusing issue. Although it appears fairly simple on the surface, several questions arise as the definitions are described. Nursing personnel for the purposes of the study include those individuals under the supervision of the registered nurse and whose salary is paid from the surgery cost center. Thus, OR nurses, educators, technicians, nursing assistants, housekeepers, and nursing first assistants are included in the study. Individuals not included in the determination of nursing time are surgeons, anesthesiologists, anesthesia team members, residents, and students. Because they are not included in the nursing budget for the operating room, they should not be used to calculate the acuity level of the patient.

Suite Preparation

Suite Preparation	
Minor	1
Standard	2
Major	3
Extensive	6

The total sample mean for suite preparation nursing time was 45.96 minutes. Four levels were identified based on the distribution of patient times: minor, standard, major, and extensive. Minor suite preparation time was 15 minutes or less and received a weight of 1. Standard suite preparation included times between 16 and 30 minutes, and a weight of 2 was assigned. The range of 31 to 45 was designated as major suite preparation time with a weight of 3. The fourth level, 46 or more minutes, was labeled extensive and received a weight of 6.

In conducting the suite preparation timing studies, total nursing time was obtained by multiplying the clock time by the number of nursing personnel involved in the procedure setup. Clock time is obtained by subtracting the time at which suite prep began from the time the patient arrived in the operating room. The number of nursing personnel in the operating room includes all personnel under the direct supervision of the registered nurse who are included within the surgical unit's budget. Suite prep includes obtaining and positioning equipment and supplies required for the surgical procedure and establishing and maintaining a sterile field. The assigned weights reflect total nursing time required to set up the operating room. The resultant levels, corresponding weights, and ranges (in minutes) are listed in the table below.

Level	Weight	Ranges (minutes)
Minor	1	15 or less
Standard	2	16–30
Major	3	31–45
Extensive	6	46 or greater

For instance, timing for suite preparation for patient A. might be calculated as follows:

    Time patient arrives in the OR 7:15
    – Time suite prep began   – 7:05
                                       10 minutes
10 minutes x 2 nursing personnel (2 RN's)
20 minutes of nursing time

Based on 20 minutes of total nursing time, the suite prep would be classified as Standard, with a weight of 2 because the range for Standard is 16–30 minutes

Or suite prep could be calculated as such for patient B:

    Time patient arrives in the OR 11:30
    – Time suite prep began   – 11:10
                                       20 minutes

20 minutes x 2 nursing personnel (1 Tech and 1 RN) plus the addition of one other nurse who assisted for 10 minutes in getting the equipment ready.

      20 minutes x 2 = 40 minutes
  plus 10 minutes x 1 = 10 minutes
                      50 minutes of nursing time

Based on 50 minutes total nursing time, the suite prep would be classified as Extensive with a weight of 6 as the range because Extensive is 46 or more minutes.

PATIENT PREPARATION

Patient Preparation	
Minor	2
Standard	3
Major	5
Extensive I	7
Extensive II	14

Five levels were identified for patient preparation: minor, standard, major, extensive I, and extensive II. The total sample mean was 72.29 minutes. Minor patient preparation was 30 minutes or less and received a weight of 2. Standard level time range was 31 to 45 minutes with a weight assigned of 3. A weight of 5 was assigned to the major time level of 46 to 75 minutes. Extensive patient preparation time was divided into two levels. Extensive I range was 76 to 105 minutes and Extensive II was 106 minutes or greater. Weights of 7 and 14 were assigned to these two levels respectively.

Patient preparation is determined by multiplying the length of time required to prepare the patient by the number of nursing personnel involved. Clock time includes the time from when the patient arrives in the OR until the incision is made. Patient preparation includes such activities as reconfirming the patient's identity, reconfirming the surgical procedure, establishing congruency with the patient's surgical consent form, preparing the incision site, providing emotional support, ensuring the patient's comfort and safety, assisting with induction, creating and maintaining a sterile field, and monitoring the environment (eg, for noise and traffic control).

Different levels, corresponding weights, and ranges (in minutes) are listed in the following table:

Level	Weight	Ranges (minutes)
Minor	2	30 or less
Standard	3	31–45
Major	5	46–75
Extensive I	7	76–105
Extensive II	14	106 or greater

For instance, timing for patient preparation for patient A. might be calculated as follows:

    Time incision made   7:45
    – Time patient in OR   – 7:15
                                   :30

30 minutes x 2 nursing personnel (2 RN's)
30 minutes x 2 = 60 minutes of nursing time

Based on 60 minutes of total nursing time, the patient prep would be classified as Major, with a weight of 5 as the range because Major is 46 to 76 minutes.

Or patient prep could be calculated as such for patient B:

    Time incision made   12:30
    – Time patient in OR   – 11:30
                                   1:00

1:00 hour = 60 minutes

60 minutes x 2 nursing personnel (1 Tech and 1 RN)
60 minutes x 2 = 120 minutes of nursing time

Based on 120 minutes of total nursing time, the patient prep would be classified as Extensive II with a weight of 14 as the range for Extensive II is 106 or more minutes.

SURGICAL PROCEDURE

Surgical Procedure	
Minor	4
Standard	7
Major	12
Extensive I	20
Extensive II	33
Extensive III	58

Surgical procedure was defined to include all nursing activities that occurred during the surgical procedure and all nursing activities that occurred until the time the patient leaves the operating room. Clock time begins when the incision is made and ends when the patient leaves the OR. Six levels were established to accommodate the wide range of times obtained in the study. These levels and weights were: Minor, weight 4 with a range of 60 minutes or less; Standard, weight 7 with a range of 61 to 105 minutes; Major, weight 12 ranging from 106 to 180 minutes; Extensive I, weight 20 ranging from 181 to 300 minutes; Extensive II, weight 33 ranging from 301 to 495 minutes; and Extensive II, weight 58 with a range of 496 or more minutes. The surgical procedure indicator is calculated in total nursing time. It is obtained by multiplying the length of time from incision to the time the patient leaves the operating room, by the number of nursing personnel involved. The assigned weights reflect total nursing time. Different levels, corresponding weights, and ranges (in minutes) are listed in the table below:

Level	Weight	Ranges (minutes)
Minor	4	60 or less
Standard	7	61–105
Major	12	106–180
Extensive I	20	181–300
Extensive II	33	301–495
Extensive III	58	496 or greater

For instance, timing a surgical procedure for patient A. might be calculated as follows:

```
Time patient leaves OR      9:23
- Time incision made       - 7:45
                            1:38
```

One hour and 38 minutes (1:38 is equal to 98 minutes.
(60 minutes plus 38 minutes = 98 minutes).
98 minutes x 2 nursing personnel (2 RN's)
98 minutes x 2 = 196 minutes of nursing time

Based on 196 minutes of total nursing time, the surgical procedure would be classified as Extensive I, with a weight of 20 as the range because Extensive I is 181 to 300 minutes.

Or the surgical procedure could be calculated as such for patient B:

```
Time patient leaves OR     14:03
- Time incision made      - 12:30
                            1:33
```

One hour and 33 minutes (1:33) is equal to 93 minutes.
(60 minutes plus 33 minutes = 93 minutes)
93 minutes x 2 nursing personnel (1 Tech and 1 RN)
93 minutes x 2 = 186 minutes of nursing time.

Based on 186 minutes of total nursing time, the surgical procedure would be classified as Extensive I with a weight of 20 as the range because Extensive I is 181 to 300 minutes.

SUITE CLEAN UP

Suite Clean Up	
Standard	1
Major	2
Extensive	4

Three time levels of suite clean up were identified: standard, major, and extensive. Weights of 1, 2, and 4 were assigned respectively. Review of the clean up times and associated surgical procedures revealed the following information. Major clean up times, 16 to 30 minutes, were usually associated with surgical procedures that required specialized equipment and/or had moderate blood or body fluid spillage (eg, micro or hand surgery, all major cardiovascular surgeries, laminectomies, mastectomies, cases requiring double setups). Standard clean up times, 15 minutes or less, were associated with minimal equipment and/or minimal loss of blood and body fluids (eg, herniorrhaphy, cholecystectomy, hysterectomy). Extensive clean up, 31 minutes or more, usually was associated with major emergency surgery, extensive radical surgery, or situational events (eg, six or more sets or instruments, abdominal perineal resection).

Level	Weight	Ranges (minutes)
Standard	1	15 or less
Major	2	16–30
Extensive	4	31 or greater

For instance, timing for suite clean up for patient A. might be calculated as follows:

Time suite clean up complete   9:45
− Time patient leaves OR   − 9:23
                                 :22

22 minutes x 2 nursing personnel (2 RN's)
22 minutes x 2 = 44 minutes of nursing time

Based on 44 minutes of total nursing time, the suite clean up would be classified as Extensive with a weight of 4 as the range because Extensive is 31 or more minutes.

Or suite clean up could be calculated as such for patient B:

Time suite clean up complete   14:45
− Time patient leaves OR   − 14:03
                                 :42

42 minutes x 2 nursing personnel (1 Tech and 1 Nursing Assistant)
42 minutes x 2 = 84 minutes of nursing time.

Based on 84 minutes of total nursing time, the suite clean up would be classified as Extensive with a weight of 4 because the range for Extensive is 31 or more minutes.

INTRAOPERATIVE ACUITY CATEGORIES

Intraoperative Acuity Categories	
Total Intra op score _____	
Circle one:	
8	Category I
9 to 20	Category II
21 to 29	Category III
30 to 44	Category IV
45 to 64	Category V
65+	Category VI

Intraoperative nursing time mean was 359.82 minutes with a range of 1702.0 minutes. Six acuity categories were established based on the total sample distribution of times. Each category, except Category I, was assigned a range by weight. A patient acuity score was determined by summing the weights (units) recorded for the four intraoperative indicators. The acuity categories and their associated ranges of units were: Category I, 8 units, 120 minutes; Category II, 9 to 20 units, range of 135 to 300 minutes; Category III, 21 to 29 units, range of 315 to 435 minutes; Category IV, 30 to 44 units, range of 450 to 660 minutes; Category V, 45 to 64 units, range of 675 to 960 minutes; and Category VI, 65 or more units, range of 975 or more minutes. Again, this was based on the intraoperative calculation that one unit equals 15 minutes.

Level	Weight (units)	Ranges (minutes)
Category I	8	120
Category II	9–20	135–300
Category III	21–29	315–435
Category IV	30–44	450–660
Category V	45–64	675–960
Category VI	65 or greater	975 or greater

Using the previous examples as determinates for the four indicator weights, the following acuity categories can be determined.

These examples illustrate how procedures of approximately the same length but different suite prep and patient prep weights can fall into the same acuity categories. The major determinants of acuity will be the length of nursing time spent in the preparation, the procedure, and suite cleanup for each patient multiplied by the number of personnel utilized.

	Patient A Indicator Weights	Patient B Indicator Weights
Suite prep	2	6
Patient prep	5	14
Surgical procedure	20	20
Suite clean up	4	4
Total Intraoperative Score	31	44
Category	IV	IV

Common Problems in Computation

The most common source of error in calculating nursing time occurs when subtracting the hours. The errors, for the most part, are due to forgetting that one hour is equal to 60 minutes, and when borrowing, units of ten are not appropriate.

Example #1

Patient preparation: <u>Incorrect</u> Way
    Time incision made   8:00
    – <u>Time patient in OR</u>   – 7:26
                                        :74
74 minutes x 2 nursing personnel (2 RN's)
74 minutes x 2 = 148 minutes of nursing time

Calculated incorrectly, the patient would be classified as Extensive II, weight of 14 with a range of 106 or more minutes, instead or correctly as Major, weight of 5, with a range of 46 to 75 minutes.

Example #1

Patient preparation: <u>Correct</u> Way
    Time incision made   7:60
    – <u>Time patient in OR</u>   – 7:26
                                        :34
34 minutes x 2 nursing personnel (2 RN's)
34 minutes x 2 = 68 minutes of nursing time

Example #2

Surgical Procedure: <u>Incorrect</u> Way
    Time patient leaves OR   11:25
    – <u>Time incision made</u>   – 8:00
                                     3:25
325 minutes x 2 nursing personnel (2 RN's)
325 minutes x 2 = 650 minutes of nursing time

Calculated incorrectly, the patient would be classified as Extensive III, weight of 58 with a range or 496 or more minutes, instead of correctly as Extensive II, weight of 33 with a range of 301 to 495 minutes.

Example #2

Surgical Procedure: <u>Correct</u> Way
    Time patient leaves OR   11:25
    – <u>Time incision made</u>   – 8:00
                                     3:25

Three hours and 25 minutes
Three hours times
60 minutes   = 180 minutes
                                    + 25 minutes
                                       205 minutes
205 minutes x 2 nursing personnel (2 RN's)
205 Minutes x 2 = 410 total nursing minutes

CHAPTER 7
USEFULNESS OF THE INSTRUMENT

The AORN Patient Classification Instrument for Perioperative Nursing is a valid and reliable tool to measure direct and indirect nursing care time provided to patients in the preoperative and intraoperative phases. Other indirect nursing care components not included in the instrument are such things as staff meetings, committee work, and continuing education. However, the instrument may prove useful in the perioperative setting by assisting with staffing, budgeting/forecasting, allocating costs, and documentation.

The basis for use of the patient classification instrument may be in documentation of the patient care requirements. Documentation of nursing care according to procedure with associated costs will form the basis for staffing, budgeting/forecasting, and cost allocation. A thorough system that can determine the nursing care needs of the patient in detail will be very helpful to the nurse manager. It will be necessary in each institution to determine the amount and level of information that will be accessed from each patient scoring. It would be most helpful to record the patient admission status, patient number, procedure(s) performed, and preoperative and intraoperative acuity categories. Some institutions also will want to record the subtotal scores obtained for each of the preoperative and intraoperative indicators to provide a more detailed accounting of the patient acuity information.

Assistance with staffing is perhaps one of the major reasons for implementing the patient classification instrument. Based on the determination of patient acuity levels within each institution, and using historical data as a base, an institution could use the patient classification instrument to predict staffing needs. Utilizing patient classification can assist in matching patient requirements with nursing resources, justifying staffing patterns, and as a basis for making changes. For instance, an institution might accumulate sufficient data to identify the following surgical procedures and their respective acuity categories.

Surgical Procedure	Acuity Category Preoperative	Intraoperative
Breast biopsy	I	I
Hysterectomy	II	III
Arthroscopy	II	IV
Lumbar laminectomy	III	V
Septoplasty	I	III
Abdominal aortic aneurysm	III	VI
Cystoscopy	II	II
Cataract	II	III

After the acuity categories are determined for a select number of surgical cases, the staff needed to complete each procedure then determine the calcutation. For instance, it may become evident that in the Preoperative Acuity Category of I, one nursing personnel per patient is sufficient and that patients can be cared for in a ratio of three per hour if their acuity is I. It may become evident that for Preoperative Acuity Category of II, one nursing per patient is still sufficient but the care ration is two patients per hour. It may be determined that the Preoperative Acuity Category of II requires one nurse but the care ratio is only one patient per hour. Based on a review of the next day's schedule, the nursing manager could make staffing assignments based on the predicted acuity of the population. If several patients were predicted for acuity category III, the nurse manager may supplement the staffing with additional nursing personnel. The same scenario can be carried out in the intraoperative phase to predict staffing needs.

The implementation of the acuity tool also can be used retrospectively to determine why the staffing was inadequate or excessive to meet the departmental demands. A comparison of predicted staffing needs based on the predicted acuity with the actual staffing needs based on the actual acuity can explain and justify deviations.

Following a thorough review of the data collected, the nurse manager also may use the classification data to justify additions to staff, changes in staffing mix, and/or reductions in staff. Most nurse managers are aware of the changes within their departmental case mix when acuity has increased either slowly or dramatically. The acuity classification can assist the nurse manager by supplementing the "instinct" with hard data. For instance, most nurse managers realize that the addition of 10 emergencies to the OR schedule within three days can cause serious staff shortages. However, convincing administration of the reasons why the department is over budget may not be easily done if the total case load did not increase dramatically during the same time. By having established a baseline average acuity for the department, deviations that significantly increase the acuity and, therefore, the staffing needs can be justified.

The classification instrument also can be used to predict patient care needs for the next budget year. Using historical data, in conjunction with proposed case load changes for the coming year, the nurse manager could extrapolate the number of nursing personnel needed to adequately supply the department. For instance, if a new orthopedic surgeon will be joining the hospital and bringing an estimated increase of 156 major orthopedic cases to the facility, the nurse manager could use the projected increase in patient acuity to project the need for an increase in staff on the orthopedic team.

The classification instrument can assist managers in determining the skill mix necessary for each procedure as well. By careful review of the acuity data, the nurse manager should be able to match the skill levels of the individuals providing care with the needs of the patient population served.

Allocating costs per patient has become increasingly important with the advent of DRGs. The majority of facilities include the cost of nursing care in the total cost for the use of the facility. The patient classification system will provide a mechanism to allocate direct nursing costs to each patient. For instance, it may be determined that a patient with a preoperative category of II and an intraoperative category of III results in direct nursing costs of $950.00. Based on this data, the nurse manager may begin to build into the costs of the procedure the costs of direct nursing care. It would be wise for the nurse manager to calculate the costs of other indirect nursing time and allow for reimbursement of those costs within the patient bill as well.

CHAPTER 8
SUMMARY

Implementation of the patient classification instrument will assist nurse managers in many ways. It will serve as a basis for documentation to assist in staffing, budgeting/forecasting, and allocating costs. Implementation of the tool will require an investment of time to review, become familiar with, and educate staff on how to implement the instrument and the benefits to the staff and the department for doing so. The energy invested in implementation of the instrument will ensure that staff are well acquainted with the instrument and need not spend more than three to five minutes to complete the instrument. Addition and final scoring can be completed by clerks or computer. The investment in money will include staff time necessary to learn the intricacies of the tool and the dollars allocated to making the information useful to the facility. Thorough investigation of each of these areas with well organized methods to implement the instrument will be a must.

AORN is committed to improving the care of the surgical patient. In this study, funded by the Association and conducted in collaboration with the University of Colorado Center for Nursing Research, the Association once again demonstrates its commitment to the perioperative practitioners and the patients whom we serve.

References

AORN research plan and priority statement. (1988) *AORN Journal*, 48 (3), 439.

AORN Standards and Recommended Practices. (1993). Denver: Association of Operating Room Nurses, Inc.

Audette, M. & Tilquin, C. (1977). Patient classification by care provided. *Dimensions in Health Service*, 9, 33–36.

Covaleski, M. (1981). The economic and professional legitimacy of nursing services. *Hospital and Health Services Administration*, 26 (5), 75–91.

Curtin, L. (1983). Determining costs of nursing services per DRG. *Nursing Management*, 14 (4), 16–20.

Drucker, P. (1974). *Management: Tasks, responsibilities, practices*. New York: Harper & Row.

Giovannetti, P. & Mayer, G. (1984). Building confidence in patient classification systems. *Nursing Management*, 15 (8), 31–34.

Giovannetti, P. (1979). Understanding patient classification systems. *Journal of Nursing Administration*, 2, 4–9.

Girard, N. & Keeler, B. (1986). A patient classification system for the OR. *AORN Journal*, 44 (2), 162–170.

Halleran, E. (1985). Nursing workload, medical diagnosis related groups and nursing diagnosis. *Research in Nursing and Health*, 8(4), 421–433.

Hart, M. (1985). An OR patient acuity system: Variable billing for surgical services. *AORN Journal*, 41 (3), 555–563.

Helmer, F., Freitas, C., & Onaha, B. (1988). Determining the required nurse staffing of an emergency department. *Journal of Emergency Nursing*, 14 (6), 352–358.

Henshaw, A. & Atwood, J. (1983). Independent nursing actions: An integral part of patient classification. *Proceedings of WSRN Communication Nursing Research Conference*. Portland, Oregon.

Higgerson, N. & Van Slyck, A. (1982). Variable billing for services: New fiscal direction for nursing care. *The Journal of Nursing Administration*, 12 (6), 20–27.

Horn, S., Buckle J., & Carver, C. (1988). Ambulatory severity index: Development of an ambulatory case mix system. *Journal of Ambulatory Care Management*, 11 (4), 53–62.

Joint Commission on Accreditation of Healthcare Organizations. (1992). *Accreditation Manual for Hospitals*. Chicago, Illinois.

McKubbin, R. (1985). Nursing costs and DRG payments. *American Journal of Nursing Administration*, 85 (12), 1353–1356.

McNeal, P., Hutelmyer, Abrami, P. (1987). Making it work right for you: Acuity recording and professional care. *Nursing Management*, 18 (10), 50-55.

Mitchell, S. (1979). Interobserver agreement, reliability, and generalizability of data collected in observational studies. *Psychological Bulletin*, 86 (2), 376–390.

Nagaprasanna, B.R. (1988). Patient classification systems: Strategies for the 1990's. *Nursing Management*, 19 (3), 105–112.

Operating Room Staffing Study. (1985). Denver: Association of Operating Room Nurses, Inc.

Parrinello, K. (1987). Accounting for patient acuity in an ambulatory surgery center. *Nursing Economics*, 5, 167–172.

Patient Classification Instrument for Perioperative Nursing, 1989. Denver: University of Colorado Health Sciences Center, Center for Nursing Research.

Reitz, J. (1985). Toward a comprehensive nursing intensity index: Part II, testing. *Nursing Management*, 20(1), 29–32.

Shirk, K, & Marion, B. (1986). Forming a patient classification system for PACU patients. *Journal of Postanesthesia Nursing*, 1, 181–190.

Sovie, M. (1985). Managing nursing resources in a constrained economic environment. *Nursing Economics*, 3 (2), 85–94.

Sovie, M. & Smith, T. (1986). Pricing the nursing product: Charging for nursing care. *Nursing Economics*, 4 (5), 216–226.

Surgical experience: A model for professional nursing practice in the OR. (1978). Denver: Association of Operating Room Nurses, Inc.

Trofino, J. (1989). JCAHO nursing standards: Nursing care hours and length of stay per diagnostic related groups: Part I. *Nursing Economics*, 4 (5), 247–251.

Van Slyck, A. (1985). Nursing service: Costing, pricing, and variable billing. In F.A. Shaffer (Ed.). *Costing out nursing: Pricing our product*. New York: National League for Nursing.

Van Slyck, A. (1987). *Report of the conference: Costing hospital nursing services*. PHS Contract (No. 240-86-0034). Washington, D.C., (NTIS No. HRP-0907082).

Vanpulte, A. (1985). Accounting for patient acuity: The nursing time dimension. *Nursing Management*, 16 (10) 27–36.

Vaughan, R., & MacLeod, V. (1980). Nurse staffing studies: No need to reinvent the wheel. *The Journal of Nursing Administration*, 10 (3), 9–15.

Verran, J. (1986). Patient classification in ambulatory care. *Nursing Economics*, 4(5), 247–251.

Whitney, J. & Killien, M. (1987). Establishing predictive validity of a patient classification system. *Nursing Management*, 18 (5), 80–86.

Williams, M. (1988). When you don't develop your own: Validation methods for patient classification systems. *Nursing Management*, 19 (3), 90–96.

ADDENDUM

AORN PATIENT CLASSIFICATION
Preoperative

Admission Status:
Outpatient, AM, Inpatient
Procedure: _____

Transport

Floor/Unit	4
Floor/Unit with monitor	8
Intensive Care unit	8
Floor/Unit special bed	12
Outpatient	0

Assessment

Routine	2
Routine with monitor	3
Extensive	4

Medications

IM injection	1 × ____ =
Add to IV bag	1 × ____ =
IV fluid administration	2 × ____ =
IV meds (push)	2 × ____ =
Eye meds	4
	Subtotal

Comfort/Safety

Secure belongings	1 × ____ =
Help change position	1 × ____ =
Assist with elimination	1 × ____ =
Emotional support (patient/family)	1 × ____ =
Constant monitoring	8
	Subtotal

Teaching

Routine re: surgery (patient or family)	1
Discharge/Home care (patient or family)	2
	Subtotal

Procedures

Skin prep: (limb)	1
Skin prep: (trunk)	2
Assist A-line	3
Assist breast measurement	3
Fetal monitoring	5
Epidural blocks	6
Axillary blocks	4
	Subtotal

Communication

Charting-add data	1
-extensive	2
Collaboration	1
	Subtotal

Patient Condition

Disability (blind, deaf, communication barrier, cognitive, foreign lang)	2

Preoperative Acuity Categories

Total Pre op score _____
Circle one:
7 or less	Category I
8 to 10	Category II
11 +	Category III

Admission Status: Circle type of patient outpatient, (AM) patient admitted day of surgery, or inpatient.

Transport: Identification of patient, determination of appropriate method of transport, and transport accomplished. Varies according to presence of patient support equipment (monitors, suctions, IV's) and location of hospital unit.

Assessment: *Routine*-History and physical, verification of procedure, review of patient record and documentation. *Routine with monitor*-Routine assessment/monitor in place. *Extensive*-Routine assessment/extensive may have monitor.

Medications: *PO, IM, IV fluids, add to IV, IV push*-Includes preparation, administration, evaluation, and charting. If more than one, multiply number by assigned weight. *Eye medications*-Includes instillation, monitoring, evaluation, and charting.

Comfort/Safety: *Secure belongings*-Assistance with undressing, identification and placement of belongings. *Help change position*-General comfort measurers (blanket, pillow, position change). Multiply by weight of 1. *Assist with elimination*-Assist to bathroom or use of bedpan/urinal. Multiply by weight of 1. *Emotional support*-Support given not accompanied by other activities. Multiply by weight of 1. *Constant monitoring*-Constant one-to-one ratio of care.

Teaching: *Routine*-Patient/family teaching including content related to surgical procedure not accompanied by other activities. *Discharge/Home Care*-Routine plus content related to discharge planning/home care.

Procedures: *Skin prep*-Preparation, skin shave, equipment disposal, and charting for preps performed on limbs/trunks. *Assist with A-line, breast measurement, fetal monitoring*-Procurement, preparation, assistance with procedure, disposal of equipment, and charting. *Epidural and axillary blocks*-Procurement, preparation, assistance with procedure, disposal of equipment, evaluation, and charting.

Communication: *Charting, additional data*-Recording additional information, beyond that associated with other activities. *Charting, extensive*-Ongoing progress notes, and additional orders. *Collaboration*-Communicating/consulting with others regarding changes in patient status/situational problems.

Patient Condition: Patients with physical or mental disability, communication barrier, and/or debilitated/frail elderly.

Version 9
4/92

AORN PATIENT CLASSIFICATION
Preoperative

Admission Status:
Outpatient, AM, Inpatient
Procedure: _____

Transport

Floor/Unit	4
Floor/Unit with monitor	8
Intensive Care unit	8
Floor/Unit special bed	12
Outpatient	0

Assessment

Routine	2
Routine with monitor	3
Extensive	4

Medications

IM injection	1 × ____ =
Add to IV bag	1 × ____ =
IV fluid administration	2 × ____ =
IV meds (push)	2 × ____ =
Eye meds	4
	Subtotal

Comfort/Safety

Secure belongings	1 × ____ =
Help change position	1 × ____ =
Assist with elimination	1 × ____ =
Emotional support (patient/family)	1 × ____ =
Constant monitoring	8
	Subtotal

Teaching

Routine re: surgery (patient or family)	1
Discharge/Home care (patient or family)	2

Procedures

Skin prep: (limb)	1
Skin prep: (trunk)	2
Assist A-line	3
Assist breast measurement	3
Fetal monitoring	5
Epidural blocks	6
Axillary blocks	4
	Subtotal

Communication

Charting-add data	1
-extensive	2
Collaboration	1
	Subtotal

Patient Condition

Disability (blind, deaf, communication barrier, cognitive, foreign lang)	2

Preoperative Acuity Categories

Total Pre op score _____
Circle one:
7 or less	Category I
8 to 10	Category II
11 +	Category III

Admission Status: Circle type of patient outpatient, (AM) patient admitted day of surgery, or inpatient.

Transport: Identification of patient, determination of appropriate method of transport, and transport accomplished. Varies according to presence of patient support equipment (monitors, suctions, IV's) and location of hospital unit.

Assessment: *Routine*-History and physical, verification of procedure, review of patient record and documentation. *Routine with monitor*-Routine assessment/monitor in place. *Extensive*-Routine assessment/extensive may have monitor.

Medications: *PO, IM, IV fluids, add to IV, IV push*- Includes preparation, administration, evaluation, and charting. If more than one, multiply number by assigned weight. *Eye medications*-Includes instillation, monitoring, evaluation, and charting.

Comfort/Safety: *Secure belongings*-Assistance with undressing, identification and placement of belongings. *Help change position*- General comfort measures (blanket, pillow, position change). Multiply by weight of 1. *Assist with elimination*-Assist to bathroom or use of bedpan/urinal. Multiply by weight of 1. *Emotional support*-Support given not accompanied by other activities. Multiply by weight of 1. *Constant monitoring*-Constant one-to-one ratio of care.

Teaching: *Routine*-Patient/family teaching including content related to surgical procedure not accompanied by other activities. *Discharge/Home Care*- Routine plus content related to discharge planning/home care.

Procedures: *Skin prep*-Preparation, skin shave, equipment disposal, and charting for preps performed on limbs/trunks. *Assist with A-line, breast measurement, fetal monitoring*-Procurement, preparation, assistance with procedure, disposal of equipment, and charting. *Epidural and axillary blocks*- Procurement, preparation, assistance with procedure, disposal of equipment, evaluation, and charting.

Communication: *Charting, additional data*- Recording additional information, beyond that associated with other activities. *Charting, extensive*-Ongoing progress notes, and additional orders. *Collaboration*-Communicating/consulting with others regarding changes in patient status/situational problems.

Patient Condition: Patients with physical or mental disability, communication barrier, and/or debilitated/frail elderly.

Version 9
4/92

AORN PATIENT CLASSIFICATION
Intraoperative

Admission Status:
Outpatient, AM, Inpatient
Procedure: _____

Suite Preparation

Level	Weight
Minor	1
Standard	2
Major	3
Extensive	6

Patient Preparation

Level	Weight
Minor	2
Standard	3
Major	5
Extensive I	7
Extensive II	14

Surgical Procedure

Level	Weight
Minor	4
Standard	7
Major	12
Extensive I	20
Extensive II	33
Extensive III	58

Suite Clean Up

Level	Weight
Standard	1
Major	2
Extensive	4

Intraoperative Acuity Categories

Total Intra op score _____
Circle one:

8	Category I
9 to 20	Category II
21 to 29	Category III
30 to 44	Category IV
45 to 64	Category V
65+	Category VI

Patient Data

Suite Preparation: Obtaining positioning equipment, establishing/maintaining a sterile field. Suite prep calculated by subtracting (-) time suite prep began from time patient arrives in OR times (x) number of nursing personnel.

Level	Weight	Ranges (minutes)
Minor	1	15 or less
Standard	2	16-30
Major	3	31-45
Extensive	6	46 or greater

Patient Preparation: Reconfirming patient identity, surgical procedure, consent; positioning; monitoring; preparing incision site; emotional support; comfort/safety; assist with induction; creating/maintaining sterile field; and monitoring the environment. Patient prep is calculated by subtracting (-) time patient arrived in OR from time incision made times (x) number of nursing personnel.

Level	Weight	Ranges (minutes)
Minor	2	30 or less
Standard	3	31-45
Major	5	46-75
Extensive I	7	76-105
Extensive II	14	106 or greater

Surgical Procedure: Total time patient is undergoing procedure. Surgical procedure calculated by subtracting (-) the incision time from the time patient leaves OR times (x) number of nursing personnel.

Level	Weight	Ranges (minutes)
Minor	4	60 or less
Standard	7	61-105
Major	12	106-180
Extensive I	20	181-300
Extensive II	33	301-495
Extensive III	58	496 or greater

Suite Clean Up: *Standard-* All activities involved in decontamination of suite, supplies and equipment requisition; and equipment transport and restocking. *Major-* Standard with specialized equipment and/or microscopes and moderate body fluid/blood spillage. *Extensive-* Standard with extensive equipment (6 or more sets), or extensive radical surgery. Suite clean up is calculated by subtracting (-) the time the patient leaves the OR from the time of completion of the suite clean up times (x) number of nursing personnel.

Level	Weight	Ranges (minutes)
Standard	1	15 or less
Major	2	16-30
Extensive	4	31 or greater

AORN PATIENT CLASSIFICATION
Intraoperative

Admission Status:
Outpatient, AM, Inpatient
Procedure: _____
_____

Suite Preparation	
Minor	1
Standard	2
Major	3
Extensive	6

Patient Preparation	
Minor	2
Standard	3
Major	5
Extensive I	7
Extensive II	14

Surgical Procedure	
Minor	4
Standard	7
Major	12
Extensive I	20
Extensive II	33
Extensive III	58

Suite Clean Up	
Standard	1
Major	2
Extensive	4

Intraoperative Acuity Categories

Total Intra op score _____
Circle one:

8	Category I
9 to 20	Category II
21 to 29	Category III
30 to 44	Category IV
45 to 64	Category V
65+	Category VI

Patient Data

Suite Preparation: Obtaining positioning equipment, establishing/maintaining a sterile field. Suite prep calculated by subtracting (-) time suite prep began from time patient arrives in OR times (x) number of nursing personnel.

Level	Weight	Ranges (minutes)
Minor	1	15 or less
Standard	2	16-30
Major	3	31-45
Extensive	6	46 or greater

Patient Preparation: Reconfirming patient identity, surgical procedure, consent; positioning; monitoring; preparing incision site; emotional support; comfort/safety; assist with induction; creating/maintaining sterile field; and monitoring the environment. Patient prep is calculated by subtracting (-) time patient arrived in OR from time incision made times (x) number of nursing personnel.

Level	Weight	Ranges (minutes)
Minor	2	30 or less
Standard	3	31-45
Major	5	46-75
Extensive I	7	76-105
Extensive II	14	106 or greater

Surgical Procedure: Total time patient is undergoing procedure. Surgical procedure calculated by subtracting (-) the incision time from the time patient leaves OR times (x) number of nursing personnel.

Level	Weight	Ranges (minutes)
Minor	4	60 or less
Standard	7	61-105
Major	12	106-180
Extensive I	20	181-300
Extensive II	33	301-495
Extensive III	58	496 or greater

Suite Clean Up: *Standard-* All activities involved in decontamination of suite, supplies and equipment requisition; and equipment transport and restocking. *Major-* Standard with specialized equipment and/or microscopes and moderate body fluid/blood spillage. *Extensive-* Standard with extensive equipment (6 or more sets), or extensive radical surgery. Suite clean up is calculated by subtracting (-) the time the patient leaves the OR from the time of completion of the suite clean up times (x) number of nursing personnel.

Level	Weight	Ranges (minutes)
Standard	1	15 or less
Major	2	16-30
Extensive	4	31 or greater